NOAH

The Best Gift Ever

a voice for everyone

NOAH

The Best Gift Ever

a voice for everyone

Written by

Laura Griesbach, M.S., CCC-SLP

ISBN:
ISBN-13: 978-1-953322-00-5

Published by Lv2Pla Publishing, an imprint of Lv2Pla, PLLC.

The author is represented by Lv2Pla, PLLC, Powhatan, VA.

Graphics designed by Paul Griesbach.

ISBN 978-1-953322-00-5

Printed in the United States of America.

LV2PLA
PUBLISHING
Powhatan, Virginia

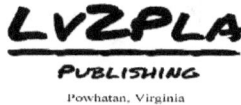

Contents

Dedication

This book is dedicated to Noah and his family.

My gift for Noah …

- To educate individuals, families, and professionals so no one else will experience what you have endured.

- To give you the words you need to say.

- To give you the last word!

My gift for Noah's family . . .

- To use the knowledge and experience Noah has led me to provide a better way.

- To transform my shock into constructive education.

- To put easy words to complex messages.

My commitment to Noah …

- To educate others so no one will say "I didn't know."

- To provide a voice for all, regardless of age or ability.

- To inspire medical and education professionals to become outraged at the "voiceless" world in which we leave so many trapped

- To provide a way for these professionals to set those isolated in that "voiceless" world free.

- and humbled enough to set them free.

Thank you, Noah for all you have shown me and for all the joy and freedom that your inspiration will bring to so many people.

Introduction

Everyone Deserves a Voice

Thank you for choosing to spend time with me and for allowing me to introduce you to Noah and a different way of helping someone who cannot find his* voice.
You will hear (or read) these words from me often:

> *Communication is a human right, not a privilege.*
> *Even those who cannot speak deserve a voice.*

That understanding and commitment guides everything that I do and is the ultimate reason I have written this book, which was a labor of love and frustration years in the making.
I imagine you are reading this because you are either:

1. a family member or caregiver for someone who is nonverbal or minimally verbal and are frustrated and discouraged with how he is treated by others and how his participation in life is so limited, or
2. a speech language pathologist or another healthcare or educational professional who wants more for their nonverbal or minimally verbal patients or students.

Either way, you've come to the right place. As a speech language pathologist, I've developed the NOAH program after three decades of clinical practice and have used it for years with excellent results.
I would like to say that technology has increased so much that nobody remains trapped within his thoughts, but I know this isn't true. I spend my time everyday focusing on all who are trapped within. Both the medical and educational models need assistance teaching professionals and caregivers how to give all people a voice.

Before we continue, I have a few disclaimers.

* The first disclaimer concerns the use of pronouns. Verb tense and noun-verb agreement gets a bit cumbersome when trying to be generic yet inclusive. So, since Noah is a man, I'm using the pronouns "he, him and his" throughout the book.

Second, I know how hectic life is caring for and working with children and adults with special needs so I'm writing each chapter to stand alone in case that is all the time you have to read in one sitting. The repetition amongst the chapters is for that purpose.

Finally, I frequently use the term nonverbal child, nonverbal communicator, nonverbal adult in order to distinguish between one who cannot speak and one who has even a few words.

There is a huge difference in the way one who cannot speak is assessed by a clinician than one who can speak. I want to drive home the importance of extinguishing the practice of diagnosing nonverbal communicators as autistic or having Alzheimer's when that is not the case. I have no intent of decreasing one's importance.

Join me on a journey as I introduce you to my friend Noah and others experiencing similar challenges. I am grateful to Noah's parents for allowing me to use his name for the program. Using his name and the acronym NOAH makes this complex process a bit easier to grasp.

Noah is a remarkable young man who inspired me to find — and now share — a better way to help those who are trapped without a way to express their thoughts or even communicate basic needs and desires. Noah's story is a classic example of how children who cannot speak are frequently treated. I will also share vignettes of others I've worked with who are trapped in their thoughts for other reasons including dementia, cerebral palsy, or stroke.

Increasing awareness and understanding of the dilemma that those who cannot speak face every day so we can change their situation is the sole purpose for my writing this book. I prefer doing therapy all day long instead of writing, but it is clear to me that my message can reach more people through a book than seeing one client or teaching one workshop at a time.

It has been so difficult to get this information transferred from my head into this book. Reading a colleague's note in a paper motivated me to finish this book.

"Don't let papers languish on your desk for lack of attention or lack of confidence" Christy Ludlow, Ph. D. CCC-SLP stated in a conference presentation. I'm guilty of both.

As we move through this book together, I will immerse you in Noah's world. I will also show you how you can make a difference for your nonverbal or minimally verbal patient, student or loved one using the NOAH assessment and treatment program that I've developed from years of working closely with Noah and his family.

Although I don't offer you a magic wand, I can speed up the process. I am here to start you on a new path by offering the gift of communication. I hope you enjoy this book and find your voice to help others find theirs!

Disney: Noah's Happy Place

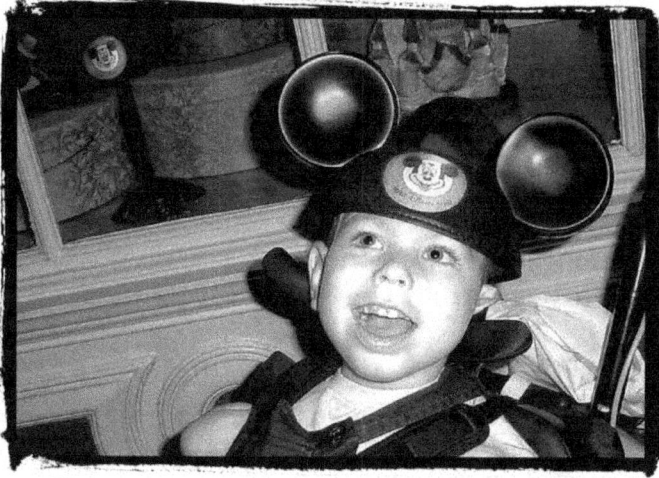

Photo courtesy of Noah's family. Edited by Paul Griesbach.

Chapter 1: Meet Noah and his namesake, NOAH

Imagine wanting to express an opinion or ask for a glass of water and not being able to get those around you to understand or even notice that you are trying to communicate.

Verbal communication is what comes naturally to the majority of humans, but over the past three decades I've met hundreds of individuals who are unable to speak. Like many of you, I am convinced that something must be done and recognize this core truth:

> *Communication is an activity of daily living (ADL).*
> *Communication is a human right, not a privilege.*
> *Even those who cannot speak deserve a voice.*
> *Intervention is essential.*

Whether you work with patients, educate students or provide care for a loved one who is nonverbal, NOAH can help you set them free from the isolation nonverbal humans face in a speaking world.

What is NOAH?

Noah is not just a what. Noah is first and foremost a who.

I first met Noah when he was six years old. I knew he was aware because during my oral motor assessment, he responded to pain with tears rolling down his cheeks as he deliberately maintained eye contact with me.

This was the only way he could communicate. He had no efficient means to communicate. He appeared to me as an empty shell, but the lights were on in his beautiful blue eyes. I knew I had to help Noah.

Today, Noah is an insightful 20-year-old who loves to communicate his thoughts laced with wit. He enjoys his family's outings, especially going to Disney World. His days involve warm interactions with his family, extended support system and the medical community. He has become quite the flirt with his young nurses. This may or may not be the reason for extended hospital visits!

So, you are probably wondering "What is NOAH?" NOAH in all caps is an acronym for a program Inspired by Noah, it stands for:

N: Nonverbal Cognitive Assessment

O: Oral Motor Intervention

A: Another Means of Communication

H: Habits for a Lifetime

Before we continue our journey with Noah and NOAH, I'd like to introduce you to a few other individuals whose dilemmas may sound familiar to you.

Trey

Lena slumped onto the floor as her husband Trey watched helplessly from his wheelchair. She wasn't responding to his attempts to verbalize. He could see she was still breathing and in pain. Fortunately, calling 911 from the house phone was a goal we had focused on during speech therapy. Agonizingly long minutes after he made the lifesaving call, he heard a knock and rolled his wheelchair to open the door. His relief was evident when he saw the paramedics on the doorstep.

Sierra

With great effort, Sierra pronounced words through her trach tube, slowly producing one word at a time. Fortunately, she was taught how to speak like this in speech therapy, so she had some way to express herself. This painstaking method of speaking would be the only way she would communicate verbally for the year before she gained her angel wings.

Mrs. Karney

"Inside." "Outside."

These were the only words Mrs. Karney could say. I'm sure these words were meaningful, but we couldn't figure out what she meant by them as she entered the late stage of dementia.

However, through observation we figured out a way to interpret her nonverbal communication attempts. As her speech pathologist, I had the honor of referring her to hospice to provide dignity for this wonderful lady.

She was 93; her husband 94. He said, "She will not live in a nursing home as long as I'm alive." She didn't have to. After we trained the professionals from hospice, they were able to interpret her nonverbal efforts to keep her comfortable with minimal challenges. Hospice helped her husband keep his promise to her and she stayed in their home of 60 years until the end.

Timmy

Timmy had cerebral palsy and was able to move about in his wheelchair. He talked at home, but not at school. At school they labeled him as "intellectually disabled" with "multiple disabilities." Advocating as a team, including Timmy and his foster mom, we ensured that Timmy was placed in his grade-level classroom with support added to manage his motor deficits related to cerebral palsy.

Why are children and adults who cannot speak presumed to have a cognitive deficit?

Mislabeling nonverbal individuals remains a problem. Children who cannot speak are labeled as autistic. Adults who cannot speak are diagnosed with dementia, specifically Alzheimer's, which refers to a change in cognition rather than a loss or lack of speech and/or language.

Consider this. We take time to understand animal behavior but for some reason we don't grant that same understanding to human beings.

Zoos, safari parks, and animal rescues, spend millions of dollars to accomplish this. In a recent visit to the local zoo, I saw so many systems engineered throughout the zoo to facilitate communication. All the animals that visitors were allowed to feed in the zoo had some engineered means available for us to do so. The giraffes, goats, and sheep could all be hand fed. The camels, rhinos, hogs, and long horned rams could be fed through PVC pipes. We could toss food down the pipe into a trough for them to eat. These animals know how to communicate with us so we will feed them.

Although we couldn't feed the tiger, I saw a sign posting information about the tiger's vocalizations. Someone took the time and expense to analyze a tiger's communication to teach others about their form of communication. There is more research out there on animals' nonverbal communication skills than humans' nonverbal communication skills.

We can, and must, do more for our fellow humans who happen to be nonverbal.

Where do we begin?

Research and evidence-based practice shows that early intervention using augmentative/alternative/alternative communication (AAC) is imperative for the nonverbal child. AAC is difficult. It is complex. It is not natural from a developmental point-of-view. We recognize that it is imperative but how do we know when and where to start? Identifying prelanguage skills is a first step.

However, when I first taught my NOAH course nationally through a continuing education provider, I was surprised to find that over 70% of the participants had no idea what was meant by "prelanguage skills." Prelanguage skills are the skills that an individual acquires before speech occurs. These skills include imitation, object permanence, comprehension or understanding, causality, a means end, and a way to have his needs met. These will be discussed in detail later in this book.

Therefore, the skills to complete **YOU CAN** of my nonverbal cognitive assessment are not well known (Chapter 4). This opened my eyes about the root cause of why many professionals do not have the experience or tools to work with those who cannot speak.

My experience in teaching the NOAH course was transformational, albeit a bit discouraging. If professionals do not know how to assess nonverbal skills or even know what prelanguage skills are, then I need to do a better job of teaching that area by spreading the message of NOAH.

My book identifies areas of weakness in the speech language pathology profession, in education, in health care and in society as a whole, which may offend some. However, my goal is to provide a step-by-step program to unlock communication for all who are unable to speak.

Too many people remain trapped within themselves, unable to speak, because of the lack of available assistance and resources. *NOAH: The Best Gift Ever – A Voice for Everyone* is a simple book to guide those who desire to change the life of another by involving them in all life has to offer.

This four-pronged systematic process sorts out your loved one's strengths and weaknesses to get him communicating *today*! My goal for this book is to reach those who need it! The NOAH program provides you with the information to know where to begin. The process I've used in writing this book is to strive to simplify complex information into a book short enough to devour within your hectic life and help you make a difference now!

What You Will Gain

Communication is an activity of daily living (ADL)! You will acquire complex, yet attainable skills to assess your loved one's cognitive and oral motor skills and then combine these strengths to develop another means to communicate. You will know how to work with your loved ones and clients to develop imitation, object permanence, understanding, causality, a means end, and way to have his needs met, also referred to as prelanguage skills.

You will help him learn to use his tongue, lips, palate, teeth, and jaws to make sounds or words, and you will provide him with a means to communicate now using Augmentative/Alternative Communication (AAC). Whether you are providing low, mid, high technology or a combination of all three, you will provide the gift of communication!

Keeping it Real

My families have enlightened and entertained me throughout my three decades as a SLP which only increases my enjoyment in my chosen profession. Noah's Dad, Keith, is one of the most entertaining without a doubt!

One session, I asked Keith and Cynthia to bring in some food to assess Noah's ability to safely accept tastes in his mouth using a net feeder. They brought in frozen maraschino cherries. Throughout the session, I'm seriously concentrating on assessing Noah's safety using the net feeder.

It wasn't until much later when I was tagged on Facebook to view the video Keith posted that I noticed something amiss. There I am, with my grape-flavored purple gloves in Noah's mouth. He has red dripping out of both sides of his mouth running down his face. If you didn't know better, it looked like I beat Noah up and blood was spilling from his mouth where my hands were placed. Thanks, Keith. You always keep me laughing!

Kinesiotape is an additional technique which you can be taught to add to your regime, to your bag of tricks. I believe therapy should be fun and so do many of my caregivers including Cynthia, Noah's mom. One of the Cynthia-driven practical jokes kept us laughing.

Noah's regular schedule meant I would treat Noah before his physical therapy session. Cynthia told me that the PT disliked colored kinesiotape being used on the face. Applying brightly colored kinesiotape to Noah's face before entering the PT room became our targeted goal. Hot pink was my personal favorite. I'm not so sure that the PT thought it was so hilarious, but I'd like to say it helped nurture Noah's witty sense of humor.

Another one of my other favorite stories happened to me when I was the clinical director of a pediatric outpatient clinic. Being the director, I had numerous other responsibilities in addition to providing treatment. One day I had an interview scheduled following a treatment session.

I completed my oral motor protocol prior to feeding one of my sweet, infant girls. On her first bite, she produced a raspberry sound with her lips spraying spaghetti all over my beige polo and white jeans. Of course, I didn't have a change of clothes with me that day. My staff loved it and enjoyed relaying the story to my interviewee. Needless to say, it was memorable. I hired this therapist. What else could I do?

High on my list of my favorite things is when families call, text, email, post, or visit me. I received a call one day from a mom to tell me how her little boy walked into the living room with *all* of the family members' toothbrushes in his mouth. She asked him, "What are you doing?" Of course, he responded with "I'm a walrus!" Walrus is one of my oral exercises. She called to "thank" me. I imagine she bought new brushes for the entire family that day.

Noah and Me at Playground

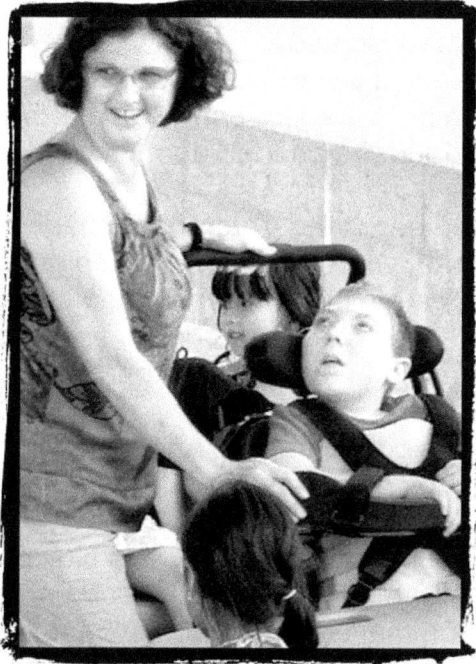

Photo courtesy of Noah's family. Edited by Paul Griesbach.

Chapter 2: Noah's Story Through My Eyes

First, some background.

I remember exactly when my passion to give the gift of communication to those who cannot speak was ignited. The summer I was fourteen opened doors for me that I never knew were locked.

I was a volunteer at the Veterans' Administration Hospital in Prescott, Arizona where my mom worked as a nurse practitioner. My mom had always shared stories from her nursing experiences in the emergency room and operating room in Phoenix and now from her inpatient hospice unit in Prescott.

Many of these conversations made it to the dinner table. There were things my sisters and I never did as a result of these stories. We were warned of all the body parts we may lose riding a jet ski, sitting on a friend's bicycle handlebars, or riding double on a bike in general. It worked because we weren't often the main character in my mom's stories. We also learned about treating others with dignity, from birth through death.

Anyway, when I was 14 a friend suggested we spend our summer volunteering at the hospital and mom made our desire a reality. I was assigned to a neurology floor. I can't recall where my friend was assigned but my experiences on that floor shaped me and those memories have never faded.

I was assigned to work with a 72-year-old gentleman who had been discovered in a camper along with his cats after suffering a severe stroke. He was so frustrated because he couldn't speak. I now know that he had verbal apraxia. Apraxia leaves many frustrated as they are unable to express even basic words, let alone sentences. I still recall the thrill and triumph.

I felt when he said his first deliberate word, besides the four-letter words he had little control over. That word was: "Laura." My name. I cried the first time he said it.

Earning my SLP and my C's

Years later, after serving five years as a Hospital Corpsman in the Navy and having a family, I earned my Master of Science degree in Speech Pathology. Finally, I was off on the adventure that I had glimpsed that summer long ago at the VA hospital in Prescott, Arizona. Little did I know then or even later as a freshly minted SLP that giving a voice to those who cannot speak would become my preferred caseload — and my enduring passion.

I credit three professors from my Speech-Language Pathology training for teaching me about the world of nonverbal cognitive assessment and treatment. Apparently, these skills are not present in all Speech-Language Pathology programs today.

Dr. Eileen Abrahamsen taught me at Old Dominion University how to assess a client's language skills, even before they learn to speak, using an informal play assessment. I shared with her recently that I still use that rough, informal play assessment form she gave me in 1988, with the same typos present. I believe it was copied on a mimeograph machine. If you are too young to know what that is, ask your grandma or great grandma. I'm only kidding about that machine, but it was before computers. I have taken that old, but essential information and embedded it within my NOAH Inventory (more about that later and where to download it to follow along easier as we continue our journey together.)

Dr. Claire Waldron mentored me after I transferred from Old Dominion University to Radford University to complete my graduate work. I observed her clinical skills in the Communication Science Disorders Clinic and wondered how I would ever perform those skills independently. Dr. Waldron was able to look at a client's communication skills regardless of age and determine if speech therapy was required. I was fortunate to be a student in her graduate level *Normal Language Development* course because she taught us the

11

higher-level language skills. This knowledge is essential to appropriately assess and treat language disorders. We limit our vision when we don't understand typical development.

Dr. Waldron supervised my graduate clinical rotations where I learned to apply my book knowledge concerning the assessment and treatment of nonverbal language skills. I continue to use those skills daily. She also gets credit for teaching me about "forms of communication" and "ranges of intention." I've been doing this for thirty years now and it never gets old. I'll elaborate on this later in this chapter.

Dr. Waldron also introduced me to the world of AAC using switches and devices many schools continue to use as their sole AAC thirty years later. She taught me about "total communication." Total communication is also called "aided language" and "multimodal". Total communication means using all means to express your needs and show understanding. Total communication strategies are what I use to get my nonverbal clients started on their journey to freedom.

Mrs. Beverly Crouse was another gem at Radford University, an instrumental clinical supervisor, who mentored me in my clinical prerequisites on my journey to become a licensed speech language pathologist. Mrs. Crouse supervised me in my very first clinical experience.

We were fortunate at Radford University to have clients with acute problems (immediately following the injury or diagnosis) and clients with chronic problems (many years past injury or diagnosis). This provided us with the opportunities to help both types of conditions. This makes a big difference when learning assessment and treatment especially for clients with neurological issues.

My first day of clinical I met an adorable three-year-old little boy whose mom unfortunately continued to drink alcohol throughout her pregnancy. "Robbie" was born with fetal alcohol syndrome. He was in foster care as he had been removed from his mother's care.

He was my first client: I was his first speech-language pathologist. Imagine his luck! With Beverly Crouse by my side, I was able to ease into his world. Although "Robbie" was receiving educational services of some type, I became his first private speech language pathologist. Through a home-based education program, Robbie had a "teacher" who used straps to tie the young child to his chair so he would pay attention to her instruction! This therapy was described as behavioral therapy!

Mrs. Crouse guided me through a process to teach this frightened child, using play therapy. I remember bringing in my daughter's Care Bears and making forts to bring him out of his shell. He began talking that semester. I learned that spontaneous language develops once a child is engaged in purposeful play. I've continued to use play as my primary means of therapy, even for adults. Now, with the graying of my hair, I can confidently say "I know what to do."

As many have said, "You have to grow old, but you don't have to grow up." I'm happy to say that I still play every day. When it came time to name my private practice, it was obvious. Lv2Pla. Love to play. It even fits on my license plate!

Now, it's time to meet Noah.

****

Noah Enters the World

Noah was six years old when his physical therapist referred him to me. His parents' sole goal was to avoid tracheostomy placement for failure to manage his own secretions.

Upon initial evaluation, Noah was barely communicative even through eye gaze or facial expressions. He was positioned securely in his wheelchair with additional support as he had minimal head control. Noah was barely interactive with people and objects in his environment. He did not use his hands at all. Noah was tube fed because he was considered unsafe to eat orally. His oral skills were weak at best; he handled his saliva by drooling or being suctioned.

Noah wasn't receiving any therapeutic or educational services except for weekly physical therapy sessions through the private agency for which I worked. He spent as much time in medical facilities as he did at home. Although his parents were strong advocates with reasonable expectations, both medical and educational intervention models of therapy for Noah were almost nonexistent. Even when Noah spent weeks in the hospital, he never received educational or therapy services. This still baffles me. He was in the hospital with the resources right there!

It wasn't like this for Noah in the beginning. Noah was born in February 2000 after an uncomplicated pregnancy. He was born at 38 weeks' gestation via cesarean section because mom's blood pressure was elevated. Noah was a big baby weighing 10 pounds, 3 ounces. His Apgar scores were 9/9. Noah "roomed in" with his parents for two days. Initial thoughts were that Noah was a healthy baby boy.

However, this perception wouldn't last long. On the second day, Noah had a seizure and was put in a special care unit for observation. All tests were normal except for mild dehydration. Doctors put Noah on phenobarbital as a precaution and sent him home. Things were okay at home for a month when "benign seizures" began. Noah continued to grow and develop until the age of 5 months. Noah was nursing, sucking a pacifier, and cooing. Noah continued to develop. He could roll from back to side and bear weight on his arms with assistance. He had minimal head control.

'All Hell Broke Loose'

Then, as his mom says, "all hell broke loose" as seizure activity increased. The neurologist diagnosed Noah with "infantile spasms" and told the family that Noah "would never be able to do anything" and sent him home.

Reluctantly, Noah's pediatrician referred Noah for early intervention services at seven or eight months old. He began physical and occupational therapy. He still did not have head control nor hand control. Noah was not aware of his hands. He did not achieve the milestone of looking at his hands as they move, a four- month level skill. I've always been intrigued by this developmental stage. This is a prerequisite for hand development. When this stage is missed so is the skill of play using your hands.

Noah was able to say early words such as "dada," "mama," "all done," etc. He was thriving as he nursed and began spoon feeding of cereal, fruits, and vegetables.

Noah's seizures increased so much that everything was tried. Stability of seizure activity and infections were difficult to manage, resulting in the decision, when he was 11-months old, to discontinue oral feeding and begin a ketogenic diet through a feeding tube. Noah has never resumed eating orally again. He continues to be treated for epilepsy, yet the seizures do not stop.

Noah continued to grow, but the relationship most of us parents enjoy with our child's pediatrician did not grow. Many things could have been done for Noah to improve his situation and support his family. The way the medical and educational communities failed Noah is an embarrassment to both professions. Noah should have received therapy services consistently, but his early intervention and outpatient physical therapy services had to be placed on hold during each hospital admission. No inpatient therapy services were ever provided. The continuum of care was nonexistent.

As Noah grew, his medical needs increased and so did his delays. He had numerous seizures daily and serious chronic respiratory infections. He received tube feedings without oral stimulation. He bounced between home, clinics, and hospitals. Noah was six years old before an ENT was willing to relieve the obstruction caused by enlarged tonsils and adenoids. He was seven or eight years old before he was evaluated by a pulmonologist as his lung functioning had rapidly decreased. Although Noah and his family were finally referred to receive medical interventions expected in the United States of America, he had severe global delays.

Noah should have received therapy to provide oral motor treatment to improve his swallowing and encourage the development of speech sounds, but he wasn't "alert enough."

15

No one knew what to do so Noah didn't qualify for speech therapy (except for my speech therapy sessions which were frequently on hold due to hospitalizations).

Noah should have received services to facilitate play skill development and self- help skills, but he couldn't control his arms. No one knew what do to do so Noah didn't qualify for occupational therapy services.

Noah should have been assessed for another way to communicate, but he couldn't activate a switch. His skills were "too low." No one knew what to do so Noah didn't qualify for assistive technology services.

Noah was too sick to stay in school so he didn't get to attend school like his peers. No one knew what to do so NOAH didn't qualify for alternatives in place for homebound students until the age of 12. Years of education and support lost because special education laws were blatantly ignored.

Noah couldn't control his head or any other large muscles of the body. He couldn't walk and realistic planning didn't opt for sitting independently or walking. Noah did have a physical therapist in his court that knew what to do. He received intermittent outpatient physical therapy, interrupted by long periods of hospitalization.

Many are Trapped

Noah isn't alone. This situation is repeated virtually every day, as those who cannot speak of all ages remain trapped in this no-man's land because no one knows what to do. They fall through the cracks — the medical, educational, and bureaucratic ravines. Consider how many people are suddenly thrust into isolation following a stroke, a head injury, or a degenerative disease such as ALS because no one knows what to do.

Like Noah, these people are cut off from their loved ones, with little hope of connecting, because no one knows what to do. I'll walk you through the entire NOAH program in the next several chapters and then, beginning with Chapter 10, I'll provide specific activities and strategies for you to use.

No One Knows What to Do

"Noah is underserved by the

medical and education models

because

no one knows what to do."

Chapter 3: Then We Knew

NOAH: The Best Gift Ever – A Voice for Everyone was created to provide a means of increasing awareness of intervention methods for those who are nonverbal for professionals, clients, families, caregivers, teachers, administrators, psychologists, early intervention providers, etc. Every therapist, educator, physician, and counselor have a caseload filled with clients who cannot speak secondary to verbal apraxia, autism, epilepsy, traumatic brain injury, cerebral palsy, dysarthria, aphasia, Parkinson's, multiple sclerosis, amyotrophic lateral sclerosis (ALS), vascular dementia, genetic syndromes, and premature birth. This list goes on and on.

Although these cases abound, training to meet the needs of these clients is virtually non-existent. As a result, these clients often go untreated because no one "knows what to do" to free them from their world of frustration and isolation. I designed the NOAH program to give you the skills and tools necessary to accurately assess and effectively treat those who cannot speak.

Provide A Voice Immediately

Instead of focusing on one concept such as speech production or AAC, the NOAH program focuses simultaneously on four interventions to address the areas of nonverbal cognitive assessment and treatment, speech production and swallowing, AAC intervention to provide a voice immediately, and daily habits to generalize these skills.

Why use a four-pronged approach? This way we are working on improving cognitive skills, language, speech production and AAC usage immediately instead of waiting for a specific level of functioning to be reached prior to giving him a voice by which to communicate.

The Goal is to Know What to Do

The goal of NOAH is to increase the number of people who "know what to do." NOAH is a systematic approach to ensure that no other nonverbal child or adult will be "under-served" by the medical and/or educational models because "no one knows what to do." To the contrary, by using the NOAH method they will "know what to do."

Habilitation and Rehabilitation take time, but *early intervention is a right, not a privilege.* Habilitation refers to helping a client learn a particular skill that hasn't previously developed and rehabilitation refers to helping the client relearn a particular skill that he had previously developed. Whether early refers to the time services are rendered after birth or after an incident, research proves that early intervention increases the chance for a desirable outcome.

Severe communication disorders affect all of us. It does not discriminate by age, gender, race, socioeconomic standing, geographical location or IQ.

In *NOAH: The Best Gift Ever – A Voice for Everyone*, you will be guided through the process of identifying goals to meet the needs of your nonverbal kids and adults who have deficits in cognition and oral motor coordination, and you will acquire components to deliver an immediate method for him to communicate.

This book is designed to be an easy-to-read book. My desire is to provide you with a no-nonsense plan to help you help your loved one and/or clients or students without the use of sophisticated search engines or a medical school library. To fully comprehend the NOAH program, please turn back a few pages if you skipped the dedication and introduction.

In addition to writing this book in which I've tried to simplify complex concepts so you can get started right away, I provide customized workshops designed to train you how to implement the NOAH program for your loved ones and clients. This isn't rocket science, but it isn't easy either, especially at first.

Noah Looking Through VR Glasses

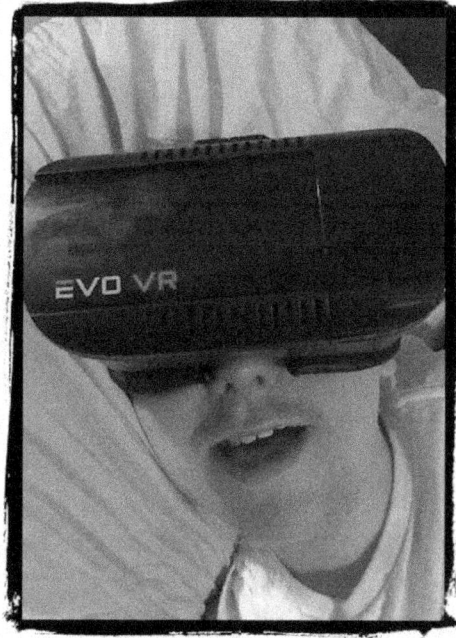

Photo courtesy of Noah's family. Edited by Paul Griesbach.

Chapter 4: NOAH: YOU CAN SEEK THEN FIND

The NOAH program is an innovative, four-pronged approach to give you the tools to help those who are unable to speak gain a voice. I developed the acronym NOAH to simplify complex information into manageable chunks to remember. These chunks are divided into two mnemonics. A mnemonic is a device or pattern of letters, ideas, or associations that assists in remembering something.

The first mnemonic spells out NOAH (Noah's name) to help you remember the big sections. As we cover NOAH, we will also explore the second mnemonic: YOU CAN SEEK THEN FIND.

An Innovative, Four-Pronged Approach
NOAH

N = Nonverbal cognitive assessment
O = Oral motor intervention
A = Another means to communicate
H = Developing habits to generalize

The letters from NOAH are the big chunks. Just as we break complex information into these four categories, I break it down further into bite-sized pieces, similar to a task analysis a teacher develops for those they are trying to teach or the steps in a recipe for those learning to cook.

To unlock communication, we need a key. Our key is the mnemonic phrase, YOU CAN SEEK THEN FIND, which makes up the step-by-step process. Unlocking communication is a complex process. Prelanguage communication must be addressed first. (I will elaborate on that in just a bit.)

The mnemonic YOU CAN SEEK THEN FIND will help you organize and apply the steps of the NOAH program.

YOU

Y = You do (Imitation/copying sounds and actions)
O = Object Permanence (the necessary skill of knowing an object exists even when the object is out of sight)
U = Understanding (directions and questions)

CAN

C = Cause-effect (action equals reaction)
A = A means to an end (using available skills to get what is needed)
N = Needs met (use of any communication to convey what is desired)

SEEK

S =Sensory (the body's response to input)
E = Examine (body posture, position, and movement)
E = Explore (mouth movement)
K = Kinesiology (muscle movement)

THEN

T = Together (who he interacts with)
H = Hierarchy (there is an order to development)
E = Engineer (create the environment)
N = Navigate (create successful opportunities)

FIND

F = Fun (communication should be fun)
I =Independent (each person has a turn)
N = Novel (communication is original)
D = Duplicate (language is naturally redundant)

These next few chapters focus on some of the philosophy and concepts central to communication development.

Chapters 10-13 will give specific activities to assess and develop the skills we discuss in the next few chapters as we explore the theory behind each element of YOU CAN SEEK THEN FIND.

As I mentioned earlier, communication is an Activity of Daily Living, known as ADLs in the rehab world.

"Communication is a right, not a mere privilege."

We all have the right to be communicated to in a manner where we can "get it." We have the right to be able to communicate our needs, thoughts and desires. Regardless of setting — home, school, group home, hospital, rehab facility, long term facility — we have the right for receptive (how I understand) and expressive (how I let you know my needs) communication.

Often expressive communication is the goal with little regard to the much-needed receptive communication. It is assumed that nonverbal kids and adults cannot understand what is being said to them. I have no idea why. Those who cannot speak do take in the verbal messages around them. They don't live in a vacuum.

The NOAH program is an original, step-by-step process to identify his strengths and develop goals to use these strengths to strengthen weakness. Instead of focusing solely on weaknesses, I find that identifying strengths is more helpful.

I strengthen weaknesses using his strengths.

I was camping recently and brought along several bags of papers that needed to be burned because they contained patient information. When I moved from my last home, the bags were packed into storage. Some of these papers were from 20+ years ago. Besides describing my procrastination and my strict adherence to handling confidential information, I do have a point to share. I brought the papers with me because it would be easier to burn them in a campfire than to shred each document.

I read each paper before I burned them just in case there was something important from 20 years ago. I saw the same scenario occur over and over. All of these test forms were blank except for the first 3-5 blocks. After that level, my clients scored no more points on the test.

Although these forms were from 20+ years ago, the scenario is the same today. There is no way to identify your loved one's strengths because the items aren't included on the test. These tests don't capture his strengths.

Yes, he has strengths! He has many strengths; they just don't ask us about them when using standardized test measures. As far back as I can recall, I write "strengths" and "weaknesses" on my test forms to engrave this information in my mind and document it in his evaluation report.

I design your loved one's therapy around his strengths, his weaknesses, not mine.

It's Not 'Noncompliance'

"If he is unable to do the task,

it is my job to figure out

what is missing;

*It is **not** noncompliance*

on his part."

Chapter 5: Nonverbal Cognitive Assessment

This chapter focuses on the "N" portion of NOAH, known as the Nonverbal Cognitive Assessment and the "YOU CAN" section of the mnemonic YOU CAN SEEK THEN FIND.

Okay, so what is a nonverbal language assessment?

Nonverbal means you can't speak.
Rarely does it mean that you don't communicate.

As humans, we communicate through the use of facial expressions, eye gaze, gestures, formal signs, vocalizations, words, etc. It would be incorrect to say that someone who is unable to speak is unable to communicate.

The important part is to assess and identify the communication skills he possesses. A nonverbal assessment is one way of figuring out what he understands and how he expresses his thoughts without speech production.

In my NOAH program, the evaluator can easily follow my mnemonic YOU CAN SEEK THEN FIND to open the doors of communication and help your loved one escape from the "trapped" world he and his family experience. With a bit of training and practice you can learn to complete the first step of the process, YOU CAN, which takes you through the nonverbal cognitive assessment, also known as the prelanguage cognitive skills assessment.

Let's briefly explore the nonverbal assessment. We will go into detail with specific activities in Chapter 10. If you haven't done so already, I recommend downloading and following along with the NOAH Inventory which is available on my website **Lv2Pla.com.** Trust me, it will make this a lot easier to comprehend and apply.

Prelanguage Skills

Prelanguage skills are the skills that are needed prior to speech and language development. English is one of the most difficult languages to learn because we add prefixes and suffixes to base words making the work more complicated. "Prelanguage" is one of those words. Pre is the prefix meaning before which is added to language changing its meaning to "before language."

All of these prelanguage skills are included in the nonverbal cognitive assessment portion of "N" of the NOAH program. You can complete the entire nonverbal cognitive assessment by completing YOU CAN on the NOAH Inventory. I will break down YOU CAN into simpler blocks.

Just as one builds a tower from Lego blocks, they combine the tiny, tiny blocks to make the big blocks work together. Ok? The tiny blocks are ***imitation, object permanence, understanding, cause effect, means end and needs met***. These skills are considered to be imperative for a child's development of language and abstract thought which we now refer to as intellectual capacity or cognition.

Jean Piaget (1952) identified these skills I refer to as prelanguage a long time ago. I won't bog you down on theory but want you to know where these come from. Let's begin to make sense of these concepts.

<u>N</u>OAH: Nonverbal Cognitive Assessment
Y = <u>Y</u>ou Do or Imitation (<u>Y</u>OU CAN SEEK THEN FIND)

You Do

"You Do" or Imitation begins the nonverbal cognitive assessment of the NOAH program. Let's begin our journey of "Prelanguage Priorities." Imitation simply means to copy. As you follow my NOAH Inventory, I'll share some facts regarding this skill. Imitation is often the skill that is missing for those who are nonverbal. It is listed first on the inventory because it fits the mnemonic YOU CAN. Prelanguage skills may develop in varying order.

"You Do" is another way of saying imitation. Before we speak, we naturally learn to imitate gestures, sounds, and speech. Imitation is a vital prelanguage cognitive skill required before he is capable of speaking even one word.

Imitation

Let's begin talking about **imitation** of sounds and gestures, then we'll talk about imitation of words. The first step to develop the skill of imitation is when a child quiets to a voice and looks at the person speaking or gesturing. This occurs by three months of age in typical language development. During the next window of development, around 6 months of age, is when a baby begins imitating sounds made by the caregiver. Even young babies attempt to copy new sounds and movements at this time.

By nine months of age, a baby imitates consonant vowel combinations. Another way of saying this is imitation of two syllable words such as dada, mama, baba (bottle). At a year of age, babies imitate single words then familiar, two syllable words or signs such as "more drink," "more eat," "daddy gone." By two years of age, toddlers imitate three syllable words such as "I love you" and speak their mind.

Don't get stuck on age levels. Focus more on imitation of sounds, gestures, or words as a strength of weakness. If your loved one is nonverbal, we need to know how to address the missing skills, not worry about age level.

Boys and girls imitate different things. My son was all about dinosaur noises, car and train sounds, and big jungle animals like the cougar. Most of these are "vowelizations" versus "verbalizations" which SLPs call nonverbal sounds because they don't contain consonants.

My girls imitated much different things. My youngest daughter played with her brother everyday with the same toys he did, but she made them "talk" using consonant sounds or verbalization vs vowel sounds only or vowelizations uttered by my son. Dinosaurs said "waa," cars said "beep," "go," and "stop." She even talked about putting gas into cars and where the cars were traveling.

My son and youngest daughter are six years apart, but that difference still showed up in my daughter's language development. Not to leave my eldest daughter out of the conversation. She came out of the womb talking and she led her brother in play in general. They are a bit over three years apart and he was led to play with toys and in games that focused on consonant production.

The presence or lack of imitation remains important to those past infancy and toddlerhood. I work with children, adolescents, and adults who struggle with communication because of progressive diseases, genetic syndromes, developmental differences, and/or brain injury from birth, disease or trauma.

The more we know about the brain, the less we truly know. It still amazes me how the brain heals! With that being said, those struggling to communicate cannot see the healing, not yet! When we talk about the act of imitation, we rely on many parts of the body to work together.

For example, your 70-year-old mom has a stroke and is now unable to speak a word. A speech language pathologist completes an assessment then gives you the results. It may sound like this… "your mom is able to understand what you are saying but is unable to say what she is trying to say." Then professionals throw out a term we learned in college and may be understood to those in the medical community, but probably not to others.

"Your mom has verbal apraxia." "What does that mean?," you ask yourself. "She can't figure out how to make the muscles of her mouth and brain work together," the SLP reports. What happens to imitation? I tell her shoes, she says "boo." I tell her table and she says "ba." Every time she says it, the word comes out differently.

Let's explore the other prelanguage skills where answers exist. As I said earlier, disease, genetics, and trauma can take away any of these prelanguage skills at any age.

Gesture Imitation

Moving on to gesture imitation. Think about a baby. A baby can imitate you and clap his hands or puts his hands up to indicate "pick me up." Between six and twelve months of age, a baby changes so much. The six-month old is more apt to imitate a sound or facial expression than an arm or hand movement but this keeps progressing so he can do both skills around twelve months.

Now let's talk about any individual who has weakness in imitation regardless of cause. What do we do? What we need to do is work on developing all prelanguage skills. Remembering that these skills max out at the two-year old level also shows us that two-year olds do a lot!

Your loved one's or client's inventory may look like this...

Prelanguage Skill	Score
You Do (Imitation)	(-) not present
Object Permanence	(+) within normal limits
Understanding	(+) within normal limits
Causality	(+) within normal limits
A Means End	(-) not present
N Needs Met	(+) within normal limits

Now let's discuss the skills of object permanence, understanding, cause effect and needs met to increase imitation and means end.

NOAH: Nonverbal Cognitive Assessment
O = Object Permanence (YOU CAN SEEK THEN FIND)

Object Permanence

Object permanence is the prelanguage skill that examines the ability to know an object exists without visualizing the object.

For the next several minutes we are talking about object permanence. What is It? Why is it important? How do I figure out if it is present? How do you help your loved one or client develop object permanence if there is a deficit here?

A child may be capable of expressing his needs by pointing, crying, grabbing or my personal favorite, biting, to request a desired object. The skills are often described as "unwanted behaviors" and a red flag for language delay. This applies to adults as well as children.

Simply put, object permanence is the skill of knowing that an object exists even when we can't see it. An object is permanent, it's always there. A ball still exists even if it has fallen to the bottom of the toy box, or in my case of my dog if Riley's ball has been purposefully hidden under the couch cushion or locked behind a closed door because we're tired of playing.

Until this skill is developed, there is no need for words. Why? Because the child can grab the object they desire without any help. If he cannot reach the object, he can successfully vocalize or use gestures to inform the other person so the object will be given to him.

For example, If I see a cookie and I want it, I don't need a word for it. I can look at it (known as eye gaze). I can point to it or I can snatch it with my hands. The problem arises when the cookie is no longer in sight. Maybe Mom hid it under a napkin, put it in her purse or closed it in the pantry.

Like all developmental skills, object permanence occurs at various ages and requires cooperation with other development skills to become functional.

Once a child is able to associate the word "cookie" with the object "cookie," he is able to request or even demand the cookie that is located in the cookie jar in the pantry. Successful communication occurs when the child says "cookie" or a verbal approximation is produced. The adult comprehends "cookie" and retrieves the delicious morsel from the jar located in the pantry."

As this scenario illustrates, object permanence is essential to language development. Potential problems can occur at any step along the way in this process. How are we able to assess if the child has the skill of object permanence? You're right, it's difficult. Too often the skill of object permanence is stagnated because of visual, hearing and/or motor impairment.

Motor and Visual Skills

Let's talk about object permanence in relationship to motor and visual skills. Since object permanence is about interacting with objects, I want him to interact with what he sees. Those skills include pulling the cloth off of his face which we see developing around six months and uncovering toys hidden by another at six to nine months. These skills lead to his removing a cover from objects invisibly hidden on his own, usually seen around eighteen months of age.

Object permanence begins with vision,
so we need to be aware of any visual impairments.

However, as instructed in the "Carolina Curriculum" don't assume a child is blind unless both eyes have been removed. Diagnoses are often incorrect or inadequate in young children or immediately after brain injury. Many adults who have vision disturbances following a stroke aren't even referred to a neuro-ophthalmologist.

Assessment of object permanence is a hide and seek challenge. Can you hide an object and get him to find it? Can they find the object whether they saw you hide it or not? You can practice these skills with your pet if you don't have a kid available. I often refer to kids, but this applies to adults too. By one year of age, a child can find an object hidden twice or behind two screens hiding the object.

One of my favorite stages of development is when a kid covers his own eyes and thinks no one can see him. Simple peek-a-boo begins by six months of age when the caregiver covers the child's face with a cloth. By two years old, a kid can find hidden objects easily. In fact, it is difficult to hide anything from him.

Auditory Localization

Another area of object permanence relates to auditory localization. Auditory localization is simply having the ability to know where the sound is coming from. This is extremely important when visual and motor impairments are present.

Some skills related to auditory localization that you'll see a kid do is to quiet down when a noise is presented. He searches for the sound and turns his head toward ear level when lying down. These skills are typically seen by three months old! Then the kid goes through levels of turning toward sound until he is able to reach in the direction of the object that has made the noise (21 months of age).

The typically developing child is able to explore their environment using their eyes, ears, hands, feet, knees, tummy, and head. Whenever there is a delay in any of these areas, your job becomes more difficult to determine whether object permanence is present, but you can through practice. You can add this skill to your "bag of tricks."

The next prelanguage skill we will discuss is "Understanding."

<u>N</u>OAH: Nonverbal Cognitive Assessment
U = <u>U</u>nderstanding (YO<u>U</u> CAN SEEK THEN FIND)

Understanding

Understanding is more frequently called auditory comprehension. Can he answer "yes/no" questions and "what" questions? Can he follow simple commands? Can he follow one- and two-step directions? ("Put it on the table." "Pick it up and put it on the table.") Can he follow "complex" directions containing things such as prepositional phrases or conditional clauses ("After we eat, we can play.")

Understanding directions is essential for structured learning and vocabulary acquisition. We begin to "know" what others are saying by first understanding their messages.

For example, once I teach him to communicate back to me when I ask yes/no questions he is able to tell me something more about his world. We didn't know that Noah was aware of his seizures until he indicated by answering yes/no questions that a suspected seizure was not a seizure, but a muscle spasm instead. I don't care what form of communication he chooses to use only that he does.

One of the biggest unintentional mistakes
that is made early on is that we stop talking to
individuals who are minimally responsive to verbal interaction.

We are totally unaware that this is happening; therefore, no guilt is allowed. He doesn't know his role in the interaction, so we often stop interacting with him – making the unresponsive individual more unresponsive.

If you are a parent reading this, do **not** take this on as parental guilt! Professionals stop responding to their less responsive clients all the time. I recently had two new students assigned to my caseload at a specialty school. One student smiled responsively to interaction and the other student did not. It's nobody's fault, but staff responded to the smiling youngster more than the other youngster.

36

I witnessed this with my eldest daughter. When she was six weeks old, she was air evacuated from a military base overseas to a children's hospital in the United States for testing. Another six-week-old baby was on the flight too for the same reason. My daughter was full term and looked like the Gerber baby with big eyes, big cheeks, and a contagious smile.

The other baby was born prematurely and struggling. This baby was adorable and sweet but too weak to smile and bat her eyes or engage others in social interaction. I hate to say this, but my daughter received most of the attention. It's just the way humans are, but I can teach you to override that natural behavior.

Noncompliance

When a client is unable to respond within the limits we desire, it often gets referred to as noncompliance. Excuse me while I get on my soapbox. This is an error in the use of the word. That is not the definition of noncompliance.

Noncompliance is to be "**defiant and resistant to authority**." That is so far off! I train professionals and caregivers almost daily in this regard.

> *"I instruct that if a client is unable to do the tasks I elicit,*
> *it is **my job** to figure out what is missing*
> *or what **I need to change** to help them*
> *to complete the task successfully."*

This is true, even if the task at hand is simply to respond to a yes/no question. Let me give you an example. I was asked to evaluate a 75-year-old gentleman who had experienced two strokes, four weeks between episodes and three months prior to my assessment.

This man was lying in bed, unresponsive to his caregivers and to me. As I completed the NOAH inventory, I found he couldn't respond to yes/no questions or follow even simple commands. In addition, he couldn't identify body parts either. I knew he had aphasia, the primary language disorder following a stroke.

I continued my assessment which includes collaborating with my colleagues and the caregivers. I asked if the physical therapist had evaluated yet and if so, were they planning on treating him. The wife's response was "he said he would see him a couple of times but would stop seeing him if he isn't more compliant."

This has nothing to do with compliance. Why isn't this noncompliance? Because the client is unable to do the task!

The happy end to this story is that I've been seeing him for five weeks now and he can follow directions, respond to questions, express his basic needs and reminisce past experiences with his wife. He still is inconsistent with following directions related to body parts in physical therapy and is gets confused upon waking whether it's day or night. What would've happened if I decided not to treat him because I determined he was noncompliant?!

As a speech language pathologist, I have a role to increase his ability to participate in therapy. Speech Pathologists take behavioral management courses specifically designed to improve a client's ability to participate in therapy so they can learn.

Communication deficits are the number one cause of unwanted behaviors, so the field of speech therapy is a great place to begin. Increasing skills for a client with cognitive and communication deficits will improve their skills in both areas. Speech therapy is a great place to begin when the need to decrease challenging behaviors is present. Speech therapy combines the specialties of communication and behavior management.

<u>N</u>OAH: Nonverbal Cognitive Assessment
C = Causality (YOU <u>C</u>AN SEEK THEN FIND)

Causality

"Is he able to cause something to happen? Causality can be difficult to assess because many of our loved ones or clients are unable to use their hands or have limited use of their hands to show us how they are able to "cause an effect."

The sad fact regarding hand use is that many therapists, educators, and caregivers don't understand their role in facilitating causality through the art of play therapy. Access needs to be provided to help those who can't activate toys and objects with their hands to develop causality. Access is simply providing a way to do something that he can't do without this adjustment. We will discuss development of accessibility later as previously noted.

Access needs to be provided to cause an effect
for those who are unable to use their fingers
to manipulate objects or press a letter on a keyboard.

<u>N</u>OAH: Nonverbal Cognitive Assessment
A = A Means End (YOU C<u>A</u>N SEEK THEN FIND)

A Means End

Is he able to indicate a way to get his needs met? Means end drives the ability to use other skills to get what he wants. A means end is not so much a temper tantrum as it is a head turn to indicate the desired drink located behind him, pulling one object to access another object, or using eye gaze to indicate someone or something is in another room.

Children with autism demonstrate mind-blowing physical
feats before learning to say the word we want them to say.

39

Means end is easy to see in toddlers with typically developing motor skills. The two-year old wants something on top of the refrigerator. They figure out how to climb onto the chair to get onto the counter and finally reach the top of the refrigerator. Many of these kids have language delays too.

Children with autism demonstrate mind-blowing physical feats before learning to say the word "cookie."

Kids with limited muscle control are able to use their muscles in their eyes more than we do. Look into their eyes for their thoughts.

Means end drives the ability to use other skills to get what he wants.

NOAH: Nonverbal Cognitive Assessment
N = Needs Met (YOU CAN SEEK THEN FIND)

Needs Met

Needs Met stands for how you express your needs. In my opinion, it is a given that over 99.9% of those unable to say a word are still able to express a communicative intent. In other words, they are able to communicate a message.

What varies is the **range** of intention and the **form** of the intention. **Range** refers to the idea. Is it a request? A comment? A label? A question? **Form** refers to how it is expressed. Crying, vocalizing, gesturing, signing, speaking, using a symbol, and/or biting or other physical behavior.

Range refers to the idea expressed.
Form refers to how the idea is expressed.

This chapter briefly summarizes the nonverbal cognitive assessment using the NOAH Inventory. Join me in a face-to-face training at a workshop or webinar to participate in a detailed training event. My website **Lv2Pla.com** provide you with the NOAH Inventory and dates of trainings.

Messy Face: The Picture Says it All!

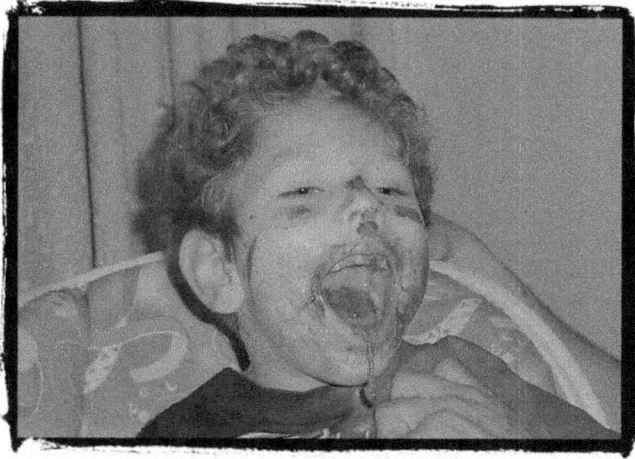

Photo courtesy of Noah's family. Edited by Paul Griesbach.

Chapter 6: Oral Motor Intervention

This chapter focuses on the "O" portion of NOAH, known as Oral Motor Invention and the "SEEK" portion of "YOU CAN SEEK THEN FIND." It is divided into two sections or blocks for easier understanding, or to take a break if you need to or have to do so.

N<u>O</u>AH: Oral Motor Intervention

Did I hear my fellow Speech Language Pathologists gasp? Why is there such a debate? Speech Pathology founders created oral motor. It dates back to 1939! If you aren't aware of the debate, I'll summarize very quickly.

The debate was created by one case study stating that oral motor intervention is ineffective for speech development because tongue strength is not a requirement for speech production.

I agree that there isn't enough university research to "prove" that oral motor intervention works because there hasn't been enough formal research, but there are numerous clinical results to lead us in that direction. That being said we need to look a little further.

There is not enough research being done to help those who cannot speak either. I've spent countless hours reviewing research for this book with minimal results found. I was impressed at a conference I just attended when one of the presenters defined evidenced based practice in a more complete way.

Evidenced based practice (EBP) is a combination of
1. review of the literature also known as published research
2. the values of the client
3. case studies

EBP is not just research alone. I totally agree with her.

*There is not enough research to help
those who cannot speak.*

*We can sit and wait for more published evidence or
we can begin speech therapy now
with what we know and what we see works*

I cannot say this enough. We can sit and wait for published research or we can start working and documenting results in a variety of ways. One of these methods is called case studies. Case studies can be technical works of science or simply stories that document the results of what you have tried. Physicians do this all the time. It works!

I prefer the latter because these stories provide me with information about what worked and what else I could have done to help me plan for my next client with a similar problem. In a sense, therapy is trial and error.

*We're in an age of evidence-based practice
being applied to direct our therapy. This is great in the areas
where research results are compiled, but very limiting in areas
that lack research.*

I'm sure the autism, apraxia, aphasia, and TBI support groups would agree that there is limited research and materials available for their loved one! Since you are reading this book, it is likely that you are searching for answers to unlock communication for your loved ones and/or clients.

43

Both families and professionals are frequently told that oral motor intervention works to help feeding skills, but not speech development. This is misleading as the muscles we use to eat and to speak have the same anatomical and physiological features.

Both speaking and swallowing also involve breath support, which is an area of oral motor skill development negatively impacted by the lack of use and/or neurological reasons.

Back to the oral motor debate. Humor me and do an exercise with me. I call it the "gummy bear experiment." Take two gummy bears or other piece of food that doesn't melt in your mouth and place them between your molars on both sides of your mouth. Yes, both sides of your mouth at the same time. Now chew the gummy bears without using your tongue at all. Keep chewing molar to molar. You're right you can't do it. Your tongue must move to allow for chewing.

I had to laugh recently when I instructed a group to do this exercise because one of the participants physically grabbed her tongue to avoid using it and to make her tongue stand still. It is difficult to keep your tongue still while eating or speaking. However, many kids and adults that are unable to speak do not move their tongue at all.

Now say the word "buttercup" three times as quickly as you can, but do not move your tongue. You can't. Now, do it one more time but faster and move your tongue this time. SLP's use this movement to assess what we call diadokinetic rate. This shows me how you move your tongue to articulate or produce rapid, sequential movements with your lips, tongue, jaw, and palate. Rapid, sequential movement is required for eating and speaking. Articulation refers to combining sounds to produce words. In school, we learn to have our clients produce "p^t^k^".

This sounds like "putaka" Yes, I get it. SLPs have a language of our own. I choose to use the word "buttercup" for him to imitate because it doesn't sound so foreign. It's actually a word. This phonetic combination provides for me as a SLP a way to assess his ability to move his tongue to all parts of the mouth in rapid succession.

*We don't know how much strength is required but we do
know you must move your tongue to speak.*

"B" is produced by pressing and holding your lips together.
"T" is produced by bringing your tongue to the top of your
mouth, "C" pronounced as "K" is made in the back of his
mouth which leads us to "P" which requires him to move his
tongue back closer to the front of his mouth so he can press
his lips together.

So how much strength is required to move your tongue
rapidly to produce those sounds? We don't know how much
strength is required, but we do know the tongue must move to
in order to produce sounds and to chew. Personally, I'm not
wasting any more time or energy on the strength issue. I'm
focusing on the movement issue, the physiological function of
the structures in the mouth. Physiologically, the tongue has to
move in various positions in the mouth even if it is only a
holding pattern.

The tongue is required to move enough to make contact
with the top of the mouth (the hard palate), the soft palate, or
the teeth to make a consonant sound. The tongue must be
able to move in a circular motion to move food around in the
mouth to form a ball we call a "bolus" to prepare for
swallowing.

The introductory exercises you learn in this book will
prepare you to teach your loved one or client ways to help
them improve their swallow and work toward consonant
production for speech.

NOAH is not a miracle program. I'm not saying, "buy this
book," "do the NOAH program then you'll speak in a week."
No, I'm providing you with meaningful ways to increase tongue
movement through repeated, structured exploration. If he
hasn't moved his tongue in fifteen years, there's still an
available plan for improvement.

It is never too late to make a change!

This change will lead to sound production and movement of
food in his mouth leading to at least pleasurable intake of food.

Once tongue movement to the palate or to the top of the mouth and teeth occurs, consonant production begins! Consonants are speech sounds which are made when the airflow is changed by the palate, lips, cheeks, teeth, or the tongue.

Once he can approximate consonant sounds, referring to consonant production without perfection, he is speaking.

Adding words together is verbal communication. I use an apraxia approach to help him learn to say each word, sound by sound, the best way he can. Then have him combine words versus waiting until a single word is pronounced perfectly. Perfection is not our goal. We can add a variety of strategies to help him make others understand the words he is trying to say.

Now let's look at the "SEEK" portion of **YOU CAN SEEK THEN FIND**. We will get to the other words in this mnemonic in the next two chapters.

N<u>O</u>AH: Oral Motor
<u>S</u> = Sensory (YOU CAN <u>S</u>EEK THEN FIND)

Sensory

Sensory refers to the body's response to tactile, auditory, visual, olfactory, proprioception, and vestibular stimuli. The sensory assessment will identify his interpretation and tolerance of receiving a message from his body.

Proper assessment of sensitivity is essential to gain sustained attention, a crucial nonverbal language skill.

I will oversimplify a complex body process. If he doesn't perceive enough response from his senses to attend to the stimulus, we refer to that as hyposensitive.

More commonly observed is hypersensitive. When he jumps in response to a sound he hears, a bright light he sees, a scent he smells or a touch he feels, or when he reacts strongly to something he tastes – these are examples of overactive response to stimuli.

Proper assessment of hyposensitive or hypersensitive response is essential to gaining sustained attention, a crucial nonverbal language skill. The body desires optimal response to stimuli to process it accurately.

To simplify this thought, it is important to know how his body responds to stimulation. More specifically for speech production is the response of stimulus to the face, mouth, and neck. If he responds more than what is expected or not enough, we will need to work on normalizing his response.

N<u>O</u>AH: Oral Motor
<u>E</u> = Examine (<u>Y</u>OU CAN S<u>E</u>EK THEN FIND)

The first "E" stands for Examine. (posture, position, and movement)

It is important to examine his whole-body posture and his ability or lack of ability to change body position. By understanding how his body is moving, we will be able to understand how his mouth is moving in desired and undesired ways. Body position begins where it is grounded, which simply means touching another surface. If he is sitting, posture begins at his bottom. If he is standing, posture begins at his feet. This even applies to crawling, if he is in a crawling position, posture begins at his hands and knees.

NO̱AH: Oral Motor
E̱ = Explore Mouth Movements (YOU CAN SEE̱K THEN FIND)
Explore

The second "E" stands for explore.

Explore the primary articulators (a fancy word for lips, tongue, teeth, palate, and jaws). These movements tell us why he is able to say certain sounds and/or why he is unable to say any consonant sounds. It also provides us with information about his ability to eat and drink.

Exploration is why boys tend to make so many sounds. Boys tend to explore these limits more than girls, resulting in non-consonant sounds. In other words, vowel sounds. These sounds are made by jungle animals, explosions, engine noises, etc. Many nonverbal kids and adults do not use their tongue or other articulators to explore movement and the subsequent sounds they could make.

NO̱AH: Oral Motor
Ḵ = Kinesiology muscle movement (YOU CAN SEEḴ THEN FIND)

Kinesiology is a fancy word for the study of how the muscles are moving. Yes, I said I was keeping this simple, but I needed a "K" for the mnemonic). It's also a good word to know. We can change muscle movements by knowing how the muscles work together. Yes, you are right. This one is a bit more confusing, but don't leave me. I will explain this in a way you can get right to work on it.

An oral mechanism examination should be completed during every speech therapy assessment and augmentative communication assessment. This information is vital to diagnose specific speech production deficits. An SLP is trained to figure out why he can't produce sounds correctly and why he substitutes or omits specific sounds.

For example, common sound errors for those trying to speak result when there is no consonant production at all. His lips, tongue, and teeth have to touch or "articulate" with another surface to produce an obstruction of airflow to make consonant sounds and they don't. It's essential to identify why he can't cause this obstruction of airflow or articulation.

Simply put, we use our lips to make the b, p, m, and w sounds. We use our tongue to make the d, t, n, s, and l sounds. We use our teeth to our lips to produce f, v, and th sounds. We use a portion of our palate to say sounds in the back of our mouth such as k, g, and h. We use the middle or front of our palate to say more complex sounds such as /sh/, /ch/, /j/ as in yellow, and /dz/ as in judge. Remember I've over simplified sound production. I use this explanation in my speech therapy sessions but provide many more details as a part of his home exercise program.

I always work on sound production regardless of his age or the length of time he has been nonverbal. I look at oral motor intervention in multiple ways. Let's spend some time on passive and active oral exercises. Active exercises are the exercises he can do by himself. Passive exercises are the exercises you need to do for him to stimulate muscle movement. Let me give you a basic protocol you can try right away.

A Simple Protocol

Before we start, it is important to mention that a professional must guide you with this protocol if your loved one has a swallowing problem. SLPs refer to this as dysphagia. I assess for these problems on a daily basis and develop safe routines for therapists, families and caregivers. That being said, if there's no dysphagia present, there's no reason you can't implement this simple protocol with your loved one.

I've been fortunate to work with Noah for many years. At one point, his Mom and I began training his nurses to complete the oral motor home exercise program I use to provide oral hygiene, passive and active oral exercises.

Although not required at all, the nurse said she needed a physician's order to do so. Therefore, we made it formal with his primary care's approval and subsequent signature.

The protocol is simple but for some reason people have a fear or unnecessary dislike of working in someone's mouth. Professionals all point to another profession to take responsibility. They claim it isn't a part of their job description. Let's end that concern now. There is not a certification for brushing teeth.

Start with Oral Hygiene

Simply take a soft toothbrush with a pea-sized or even smaller amount of toothpaste. If he is able, you can do this at the sink. If not, I bring the water to him. I like to use two separate cups filled halfway with water. Simply wet the toothbrush by dipping it in one of the cups of water. Brush his teeth like you brush your own teeth.

Rinse between brushing in the other cup of water. You will end up with a "clean" cup of water and a "dirty" cup of water. If the "dirty" water becomes too dirty, you will have to empty and refill with clean water.

With firm pressure massage his tongue with a toothbrush to remove debris. I actually prefer using the toothbrush bristles instead of the massager on the back of the head of the brush to scrape the residue off of the tongue. Avoid going too far in the back of his mouth so you don't trigger the gag reflex.

Continue rinsing the brush in the "dirty" cup and dipping in the clean cup to get a little bit more clean water to further clean the mouth. Massage the inside of the cheeks and the top of the mouth with the bristles, rinsing as you go. Thoroughly rinse his mouth.

I use very little water to decrease the need to manage the water remaining in his mouth especially if he has swallowing problems. I use 2x2 pieces of gauze to provide additional scrubbing and to absorb water. It is amazing how much water gauze absorbs. His mouth should be clean now so we can accomplish a simple oral exercise program while we are still working in his mouth.

Oral Motor Protocol

The Oral Motor Protocol I use is as follows:

1. Move the brush to the inside of his left cheek so his tongue will follow the brush to that cheek to facilitate tongue lateralization. This simply means moving his tongue to each side. If he can move his tongue independently, this is an active exercise.

   If he cannot move his tongue to the side by himself, then I will push the side of the tongue to get a reflexive type of response for the tongue to push back and then follow the brush to the left side of the mouth. This is a passive exercise. Passive is when we perform the exercise for him to encourage tongue movement. This increases his ability to explore how to make mouth movements and sounds independently. Continue to the right cheek and repeat. We will always be working up to ten repetitions on each side.

2. Next, we work on tongue protrusion, which is simply sticking your tongue straight out of your mouth without using the lips or teeth to support the tongue which is a collective group of many muscles. No, we don't stick our tongue out of our mouth to say any sounds, but this movement shows us if there is enough jaw stability for him to move his tongue side to side. SLPs call this tongue dissociation.
   If he has been determined unsafe to eat, then a professional swallowing assessment is required to develop a safe protocol for him.
   If he can stick his tongue out by himself, this is an active exercise. If he cannot, then assist as a passive exercise. I encourage tongue movement with the use of

a mirror to provide visual feedback. As a rule, kids love mirrors. Adults do not, but I still like to use mirrors if the adult will participate. I also encourage tongue protrusion by adding flavor, if possible, on the brush, or a sucker, a popsicle, and/or ice cream cone, etc.

Tongue protrusion is a complex oral motor skill. If he is unable to do this, ask for a speech therapy assessment. You will be glad you did!

3. Jaw stability is a prerequisite, or the skill he must possess before active tongue lateralization is present. You can spot this by having him stick his tongue out of his mouth and move his tongue side to side without his lips touching his tongue or teeth. If he can't do that, I teach an exercise I call walrus. (You may recall an earlier reference to this exercise with one of my young patients adapting it by using the entire family's toothbrushes.

   For walrus, simply take two craft sticks and place them between the upper and lower molars on each side of his mouth like he is biting something with his molars. Have him hold the sticks with his molars working up to ten seconds. This exercise strengthens the jaw muscles. A strong, stable jaw is required in order for him to move his tongue separately from his jaw. I also use many other professional techniques which require further training.

4. Lip closure is the final oral exercise I will provide in this book. Lip closure is a problem I see on a daily basis. One simple exercise you can do is place a craft stick flat on the lower lip. Have him close his lips together.

   I discussed in the assessment chapter that it is important to know if the top lip doesn't come down far enough to touch the bottom lip or the bottom lip doesn't come up far enough to touch the top lip. This requires a professional assessment.

Regardless, if he can bring his lips together to hold the craft stick in his mouth you will be strengthening lip closure. Have him hold the stick using both lips and work up to pressing his lips together for ten seconds.

Please note: This section is not designed to comprehensively train you in oral motor intervention, but to increase awareness and encourage him to move his oral muscles. **This basic routine is safe for him unless he has problems swallowing. Much more training is required to perform any sort of oral motor intervention in that circumstance.** However, it is quite easy to get a speech assessment for your loved one.

An online resource for oral motor intervention is the website **oralmotorinstitute.org**. This site was founded by two SLP's Pamela Marshalla and Diane Bahr in 2007 to add information and evidence base for oral sensory and oral motor techniques for articulation, motor speech, and feeding treatment. Check it out!

During my consultations, I go through a detailed swallowing assessment and design a safe oral motor intervention for him. I always do oral hygiene and exercises for every client I treat.

I provide a hands-on training in my NOAH program workshop designed for professionals and families. I educate professionals with the ability to train other professionals in my NOAH Certification Program.

The 5-year-old Gets It!

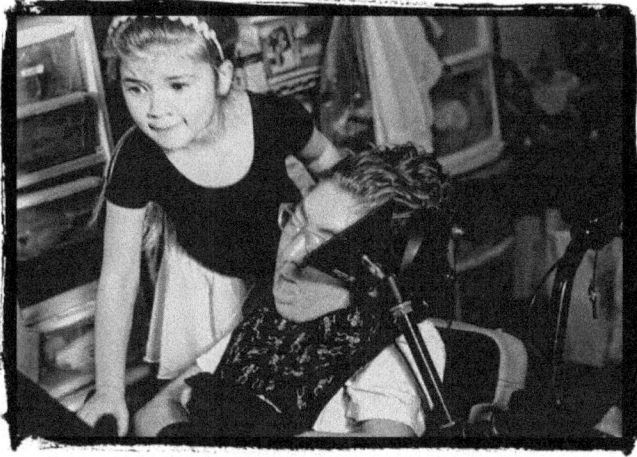

Photo courtesy of Paul Griesbach.

**Noah and his niece, Kinlee, connect
using his augmentative communication system.**

Chapter 7: A: Another Means to Communicate

This chapter focuses on the "A" portion of NOAH, "**A**nother means to communicate" and the THEN section of the mnemonic YOU CAN SEEK THEN FIND.

This is by far the most difficult chapter to write in this book. Allow me to share some information before I get to the "THEN."

The American Speech Hearing Association (ASHA) defines Augmentative and Alternative Communication (AAC) as follows: AAC includes all forms of communication (other than oral speech) that are used to express thoughts, needs, wants, and ideas.

We all use AAC when we make facial expressions, use gestures, utilize symbols or pictures, or write a message. I am frequently told that I don't have to speak a word; my face says it all. You may be told the same.

In today's high- tech world, AAC also encompasses the many devices that can be used by nonverbal or minimally verbal clients to enhance the ability to communicate. In my experience, the use of augmentative/alternative communication (AAC) is the answer to providing "another means to communicate" before he can speak clearly and efficiently.

I will refer to this means as AAC from here on. I want you to be familiar with the abbreviated expression because it is shorthand for the "A" in the mnemonic NOAH. AAC is the terminology that most of us are using now in the field of communication. Augcom is also used by some of us who have been practicing AAC for a longtime.

No Means to Express

AAC is an area in which most professionals, clients, and families have insufficient information. This arm of our four-pronged approach is essential because AAC is how we give him a voice to "augment" which means to add to his existing communication.

"Alternative" means to find another way for him to communicate when verbal skills aren't present or efficient.

I am appalled at the number of children and adults who are seen by therapists and educators but are not given a means to communicate. Kids are left to their own vices to communicate within the classroom and at home when they have no means to express their needs, ideas, and desires or demonstrate comprehension of what is taught to them. Adults are locked in their home or facility unable to express their thoughts, ideas, and experiences they've gained from a lifetime of learning.

As we discuss this complicated topic of AAC, I want you to think of a client or your loved one, just one person.

Max Benefit

Frequently, I'm asked to consult for kids and adults who once received speech therapy and who were discharged from speech therapy with the terminology "goals met" or "max benefit achieved" glaring in their reports.

> *In my opinion, it's never okay to discontinue*
> *therapy services before your client*
> *possesses a means to communicate,*
> *unless **he** chooses to discontinue treatment.*

All nonverbal individuals should be referred for an assistive technology and speech language evaluation. **No exceptions.** Sometimes these two evaluations are completed by the same speech pathologist. Some referral sources have these two assessments completed by two different therapists.

We often try to differentiate therapy by the location in which the client receives treatment. Environment should have minimal impact on the client because we must be able to communicate in all settings. Most of my clinical experience is in private practice, but most of my clients were school age; therefore, I was involved in their school programming.

In thirty years, I have purposefully worked in all settings to gain knowledge and expertise to find a better way for him to communicate 24/7, 365 days a year.

Learned Helplessness

I have worked in public school systems in addition to my private practice to observe how AAC is managed. What I have found is that public school systems are one of the most difficult settings to help students acquire AAC skills. I quickly saw the complexity of managing AAC throughout the school district.

The school is the setting where you can reach so many children because they are required to attend school. This increases the necessity to ensure that they are receiving the assistance and support for those who cannot speak clearly and efficiently.

However, most nonverbal students have no system by which to communicate. These students are dependent on school staff to interpret their nonverbal communication attempts. They either become passive non-communicators or develop learned helplessness when their attempts to communicate are not interpreted.

*People tend to speak **at** a nonverbal client
versus communicating **with** him.
Unless there are expectations that the student
has thoughts about what is being said to them,
no further communication occurs.*

Although these students receive exceptional care for their physical needs, communication is a low priority for them throughout their day at school and even in their homes for many reasons. I'm stating this objectively. I am not judging the school system, the student, caregivers, or the educators. I am simply identifying the complexity of the problem. This includes all school systems, not just the schools I've interacted within.

I focused on incorporating the NOAH program to make a change by implementing the three areas assessed:

Nonverbal cognitive assessment,

Oral motor intervention

Another Means to Communicate (**A**AC implementation).

The "H" in NOAH (**H**abits for a Lifetime) makes the first three possible for the client for the rest of his life. Insights will be described in the sequel to this book: *NOAH Goes to School.*

Now, back to the "A" in our mnemonic device NOAH. Later in this section I will walk you through the steps for the mnemonic "THEN."

NOA̲H: Another Means (to Communicate)
A = Another Means or AAC.

AAC allows you to act upon his needs immediately by providing a means to communicate. By no means will you become an expert in the field of AAC just by reading this book, but you will know what steps to take next.

"Technology changes quickly" is an understatement!   From the time you pick up this book to the time you finish it, technology changes will have occurred.

One thing that is well documented is the inconsistency of technology. One moment it works, the next it doesn't. This negatively impacts the development of communication because of inconsistency with cause effect. It may also decrease your motivation to use technology because of the troubleshooting and problem-solving accompanying technology. Some of you reading this may be saying, "I can't do this technology stuff." or "I'm not into it."

I understand and truly empathize. I can't even figure out how to use all the remote controls at home or reboot the satellite. If I were left on my own, I wouldn't have TV at all. Why can't I do all those things? Simply put, the desire to meet that need isn't present. At work, I can grab a piece of equipment and troubleshoot it successfully most of the time.

That's because the desire, the need to know, is present. I try to learn whatever is thrown at me because I am committed to the "need" that all have the right to communicate. I'm more than okay with turning the TV off!

I wish I could say, "You don't have to bother with the technology piece," but I cannot. I need you helping your client, your child, your loved one to use the available technology to help them communicate. Thank you and I will continue to help you.

I still don't feel like an expert and I use AAC daily! AAC technology is dynamic, meaning it changes and changes quickly! Technology to support AAC is ever changing regarding to access, hardware, and software. However, there are many resources available to use in conjunction with this program.

The NOAH program is not designed to be provided in isolation. My program can (and even should) be used in combination with other programs.

A Process

NOAH is a process that leads to the identification of strengths and weaknesses which provides intervention of multiple skills simultaneously. The NOAH inventory and subsequent treatment protocol can be combined with any program you are doing in school and out of school.

I don't believe in excluding other programs. My therapeutic skills have been developed to the level at which I practice because of learning about many ideas, protocols, and practices. One alone isn't enough. Combination is key. Please combine the NOAH program with other techniques you may be using or will learn in the future.

Now that we've covered the "A" of the NOAH program, let's talk about ways to implement it, to set communication in place for those who cannot speak, cannot be understood or are not efficient with verbal communication. In other words, let's talk about "THEN", the next portion of YOU CAN SEEK THEN FIND.

"THEN" describes how to both assess and implement AAC into his environment.

Let's dig into the details of "THEN" because the use of AAC is so misunderstood. Simply put, AAC is developing a way to express himself. Remember, the first "A" stands for "augmentative," which means to add to what he already uses to communicate: gestures, signs, facial expressions, eye gaze, words, pictures, symbols, etc. We don't extinguish these means to communicate. We **add** AAC strategies to help him communicate clearly and effectively.

The second A stands for "alternative." When he has no consistent ways to communicate, we must develop a means to do this *now*. It's important to provide an alternative way to communicate. This is when he is unable to speak — truly nonverbal. In this case, he needs an alternative means to communicate such as a speech-generated device which permits access to thousands of words. These devices provide a system to fully access language.

I cannot stress enough how important it is to provide an alternative way to communicate. I'll be honest, this development is a trial-and-error process. There are so many ways to do this effectively. Please don't be afraid to put something together and totally change your mind six weeks later. I do it all the time! It is important to document the "trialed" system, so you don't throw the baby out with the bath water before selecting a new avenue to communication.

Of course, I do have my favorite companies and devices that I prefer, but new systems are developed all the time.

NOAH: Another Means (to communicate)
T = Together (YOU CAN SEEK THEN FIND)

Together

A communication inventory will identify who he interacts with. It is important for him to interact with other people than just his immediate family and medical/educational professionals. Who is in his life?

Far too often, the only people involved in his interactions are either his family and the AAC user or his teacher and/or therapist and the AAC user. We need to include everyone in his life. "Together" includes parent/guardians, siblings, spouse, friends, relatives, professionals and acquaintances.

Many books include some of these people, but not all of them. I like *Social Networks: A Communication Inventory for Individuals with Complex Needs and Their Communication Partners.* Blackstone, Sarah W., Ph.D., Berg, Mary Hunt, Ph.D. Copyright 2003., Augmentative Communication, Inc.

Social Networks was designed to help providers establish and realize goals that enable individuals with complex communication needs to interact with the people around them. *Social Networks* added the concept of acquaintances in their plan. Acquaintances are defined as people we don't know. This category is helpful to teach both stranger awareness and opportunities to increase interaction with people we don't know. We eventually need both groups in our daily activities for functional, meaningful communication.

Another great resource is *Circle of Friends*, which was developed in 1989 by Marsha Forest and Judith Snow. This idea was developed to promote inclusion in the classroom. I used this as a tool in my social groups in the 90's. It remains effective today in my practice.

The NOAH inventory will identify who he has opportunities to interact with. It is important for him to interact with people other than just the immediate family and medical/educational professionals.

One of my favorite clients I worked with was a woman in her eighties. She survived a complex stroke and was left with severe verbal apraxia. She knew exactly what she wanted to say, but it wouldn't come out clearly.

In my therapy sessions, I like to develop a list of who's who in their family to establish who "together" is in the family. This increases the chance he can initiate conversation with family members by name. If the client can't pronounce them by name, I include the name in the AAC system.

This woman's name was Leah it is fairly easy to say but, of course, it wouldn't come out clearly for her. What tickled me was that many members of the family had her name — either as a first or middle name. By the time we finished our "together" list, we were crying from laughing so hard! I do try to encourage humor to alleviate the pain and frustration of the situation.

There is a good end to this story. Thankfully, she was able to regain her ability to pronounce her name and all those family members who shared her name. She regained this skill just as her great, great granddaughter was born who also shared her name. Yes, we laughed about that too! The point is to include the entire team as part of "Together" as described on the NOAH inventory.

Continue with me as we discuss the details of **"H"** in the mnemonic **"THEN."**

NOAH: Another Means (to communicate)
H = Hierarchy (YOU CAN SEEK THEN FIND)

Hierarchy

For our purpose, **hierarchy** refers to the order in which AAC skills are developed. There are three levels of AAC users most commonly described.

Level one, emerging, is when he is first exposed and beginning to use AAC. The second level is context dependent. He requires contextual cues and prompts to use the system he is familiar with. The third level is independent.

I rarely get to see an AAC user at the third level because I'm usually the SLP initiating AAC. This level is nothing short of amazing to me! It means the AAC user has been using his device(s) and can now hold his own in conversation. You find evidence that early intervention is almost always present when you see this success. I would see this level of communication more frequently if more people become familiar with using AAC.

Low technology options should be used immediately
while pre-language skills are being developed.
Keep in mind that this has nothing to do
with chronological age or intellect.

How can we increase independent communication without some form of communication? A toddler who isn't speaking or isn't speaking clearly enough to be understood can hit a switch to take his turn in a social game by saying "more," "it's my turn," "will you play with me?," or repeating a phrase in a song or book such as "run, run as fast as you can; you can't catch me I'm the Gingerbread man!"

All of this information is beneficial to include in the AAC evaluation. The SLP writes the augmentative communication report in order to purchase an AAC system, known as a speech-generated device.

Children and adults receive personally prescribed wheelchairs and other adaptive equipment, but communication systems are looked at differently by many people. Can you imagine if a student showed up at school without a personalized wheelchair? In reality, AAC is simply another piece of durable medical equipment to achieve an ADL, an activity of daily living. This is his voice!

Moving along in our mnemonic THEN, **with** the letter "E."

NOAH: Another Means (to communicate)
E = Engineer (YOU CAN SEEK THEN FIND)

Engineer
"E" stands for Engineer. It is important to create an environment to facilitate communication. To be able to anticipate communication needs that arise require excellent observational skills and the patience to take that time. Keep in mind the concepts of form and range of communication intentions discussed in chapter one under "**N**" in the nonverbal assessment portion.

Engineer isn't my term but it's a good one. The verb form of engineer means to design or build a machine or structure. It takes effort to design or build a communication system. It's hard to make it simple. Keep in mind that there isn't only one way to build a successful system. I try to let those using the system build it. If they are unsure, I'll help them, but I want them to work on creating the system. Who is "them?" All the people you listed on the "together" step equals "them." Expect changes to his system. Change is growth. Finding the best system is trial and error. Most importantly, there are many end results with equal success! There is more than just one way to do it right!

Finding Normal

Using multiple communication systems is the norm. Even when he uses a high-tech speech generated device, he needs access to a picture system as a backup.

As mentioned before, I never feel like an expert with AAC because of the constant changes in technology. I'm not even an expert with my personal cell phone and it's ever-changing capabilities.

Working with clients, families, and educators to develop successful systems requires listening, time, analyzing, and patience with technology. Only one goal is required. The goal is to provide an effective communication system for the client.

What determines it to be an "effective system" varies from client to client. That's it! It doesn't matter if the system is low tech, mid tech, high tech, or a combination thereof, but the ability to successfully use the system or systems is the ultimate goal.

Let's talk about the difference between low, mid, and high technology. Low tech refers to the use of pictures used individually or arranged in a system that is non-electronic. This is usually the first AAC system introduced and the back-up system for higher tech devices.

Mid-tech is an electronic means of communication, but not a computer. These AAC devices tend to have a grid where pictures and icons are available for the individual to select from a few to many pictures, symbols, or words.

High-tech is an electronic means of communication which is essentially a computer or tablet. These AAC devices provide a dynamic display with thousands of word and message options to access communication. The software is a complete communication system.

An AAC assessment, performed and written by an SLP, is required to purchase a communication device. A team approach is highly recommended when assessing a client for an AAC device. Keep in mind that the SLP is required to write the report to obtain funding by most insurance companies.

There is so much support out there to help you accomplish this. Do **not** be afraid to order a dedicated communication device. You will open a new world for him. Keep in mind that the device you order should meet his needs for five years because that's how long before most insurance companies will pay for a new device.

Communication is a treasured gift to provide for anyone trapped within their thoughts! We are teaching how to communicate, not how to use a device.

Strengths to Strengthen Weaknesses

Regardless of the diagnosis, all pieces of the puzzle need to be identified. I refer to these as strengths and weaknesses. The first thing I do when I begin working with a client is to complete the NOAH inventory so I know his strengths and weaknesses. **"Identifying Strengths to Strengthen Weaknesses"** has been my catch phrase for decades.

For example, when I begin working with a client who is currently verbal, but is losing his ability to speak due to a degenerative disease or process, I add the high technology piece immediately so they learn how to use it before they need it. Low-tech can be put in place immediately with mid-tech used as well.

I worked with a gentleman with a rare brain disease that was stealing his ability to speak. His cognitive and language skills were superior. He was a professional working in the field of rehabilitation which made the situation even sadder and the urgency on my part to ensure he could communicate. Initially, he used AAC to maintain his ability to work. Eventually, he used AAC to communicate his final wishes.

The way we engineered his environment wasn't to build language skills, but to keep a means to communicate available as his speech production deteriorated. High level language skills were already present.

Initially, a high-tech device was ordered to teach him how to use it when he needed it. This allowed him to keep up with professional speeches and conversations within his professional and personal worlds. He used his phone to augment his speech as his speech intelligibility decreased.

Finally, another device was added as technology caught up providing him with a portable high-tech device to replace the larger cumbersome device. His entire day was engineered to meet his needs and keep communication open as his disease progressed. Planning for his day was required.

Our society is all about technology. As I research AAC technology to simplify the "A" in NOAH, it is blatantly obvious how complex it has all become. Hardware and software are two words I rarely used until recent years, but I find myself using these terms daily. We will discuss hardware and software in addition to more on low, mid, and high technology in Chapter 9, the Step-by-Step chapter.

NOAH: Another Means (to communicate)
N Navigate (YOU CAN SEEK THEN FIND)

Navigate

Navigation in this context means to create successful opportunities to use technology to direct, manage, and communicate. By creating opportunities to communicate, he can learn how to initiate conversation, respond to conversation, take verbal turns in conversation to maintain the topic, and end the conversation. He will learn to manage his communication by identifying and repairing failed communication attempts. This is a requirement in communication in general, not specific for AAC users.

Navigation. What does this have to do with helping someone speak? When my family travels, the person who sits shotgun is the Navigator. Regardless of age, if you take that seat you get to direct, manage, and communicate. There are times I will take the back seat literally because I don't want the role of the navigator. I specifically choose not to direct, manage, nor communicate. There is a lot of responsibility as the navigator.

When I was a kid, we used AAA Triptiks on long trips. I loved it! I remember navigating as a young child from the back of the family station wagon. My dad liked to drive at night on our trips from Arizona to Virginia and back. I'm a night owl so I "drove" with him until I eventually joined my sisters in slumber.

A Triptik allowed you to direct the driver before the interaction occurred. Of course, today's travel is navigated by GPS, but she has to recalculate frequently. She doesn't take her role of navigation seriously! On the road, navigation means directing the driver to take action before you miss the turn. For speech and language skills, this means figuring out how to apply all the communication accommodations that he requires just like you are adjusting for visual, hearing, and/or motoric impairments.

Managing as the navigator means juggling things. The navigator manages the GPS, maps, cell phone, snacks, drinks, the music playing in the car, and even the conversation in the car. Sometimes the navigator tells everyone in the car to be quiet so he can do his job!

Managing the conversation as the navigator requires choosing the desired communication system(s) that he uses. Sometimes it requires the AAC user telling people to be quiet so he can focus or assisting the staff or family members to use the AAC system to communicate a message.

Now that we've completed "THEN," let's look at some examples that illustrate how different this can look from individual to individual.

One Fall, I assessed each student in a class of four students. Each student exhibited different needs, especially in the area of communication. I had to take into account what the teacher and parents were comfortable doing as well. After assessing the teacher's students, this is what I came up with to trial in September.

Student #1

Student is able to speak with adequate intelligibility by those familiar listening to her. She requires activities which encourage her to use her current vocabulary while being exposed to new vocabulary daily and encourage repetition of this vocabulary. She needs a variety of technological support to augment the vocabulary she is currently using. This can be in the form of any level of technological support; however, vocabulary selection is essential to her progress.

She needs the vocabulary to improve the form by which she communicates her intentions. Remember the discussion about form and intention from chapter 5? Currently, she fills the gaps in her communication by sticking her tongue out or swatting at people within hitting range. Adding vocabulary to engage her in topic starters will allow her to communicate with success and decrease behaviors such as hitting others or sticking her tongue out at them.

The form may be a picture attached with Velcro or a tablet with a communication app. I've chosen to use a cell phone with a free software download right now because it's compact, available, and prepares her for a more complex device if her speech and language remain slow to develop. Technology allows the user to hear the word repeated more than you will want to repeat it. Repetition is so important. She will need to activate her device often in order to get her to use it daily.

Student #2

This student is unable to speak but vocalizes and uses eye gaze with pictures consistently. He is able to activate a switch with his hand with effort. He is ready for a speech generated device. However, he's never been exposed to this technology by his family or teachers.

I recommend a trial use of a switch to increase purposeful use of the switch to activate a single prerecorded message. At his age we often use vocational or "life skills" equipment to be activated by a switch. He can activate a shredder, a pencil sharpener, or a dispensing cup. This also means he can activate a computer, a fan, a mixer, a blow dryer, or have access to electronics to enjoy music or videos; however, a different system for communication is needed for immediate results.

A trial of pictures on an eye gaze frame is a step to get his family and his teacher on board with me. The use of eye gaze technology to activate a speech generated device is a realistic goal for this student. These communication systems should provide the individual with the ability to perform these three skills:
1. Ability to respond to yes and no questions (preferably using his own body parts such as his head or eyes).
2. Ability to make a choice from a minimum of a field of three.
3. Ability to retell a story or experience using 3-4 pictures. This trial should lead to AAC with a dynamic display with software with access to thousands of words.

Student #3
He is able to say several words. He has verbal apraxia. Sometimes those strings of words come out intelligibly, other times not so much. He needs augmented speech which will help him demonstrate that he knows what is going on because he does! AAC gives him the words to express his thoughts.

At this point, I don't have "buy in" from his teacher or his family so I will trial pictures to increase his ability to combine current words with pictures and written words. "Buy-in" isn't difficult to attain once the user communicates a message using AAC.

I always include words and pictures because decoding letters into words develops at all ages. If he can't speak, he can't let me know that he can already read. He needs a minimum of 3-4 pictures presented at a time to provide conversation. We discussed providing aided language.

Aided language is pointing out the symbols on the device as we use total communication. The analogy I use to explain aided language input is when you call a corporation and the automated computerized system answers your call. The computerized voice narrates the choices.

"If you want to speak to people with answers, push 1.

If you want to speak to the people without answers, push 2.

If you want to speak to disgruntled employees, push 3.

If you want sarcastic answers, push 4.

If you want a peppy voice, push 5."

Following the list of choices, it says if you need to hear the choices again, push 9. That's how aided language input works, but hopefully you have better options than an automated phone system provides.

Aided language input allows your loved one to hear all the possible choices then make a selection. For example, "Do you want to read *Harry Potter, Three Little Pigs, Tom Sawyer*, or *NOAH: The Best Gift Ever – A Voice for Everyone?*"

Aided language input provides a simple method to increase choice making. Aided language input should be used with emerging AAC users, not permanently. Speech generated devices are created for user-initiated communication. The AAC user must learn to be the initiator, not just a responder to communication messages, to become an independent AAC user.

Using eye gaze or direct select (when he pushes the button), he will look at the pictured selections as the conversation partner points to the pictures. He doesn't have to request his partner to repeat the selection, the partner automatically reads the list of choices again as he points to the pictures until he makes a selection.

Communication is not a test! He hasn't lived in a vacuum. He hears the words around him. He understands what is being said around him. You don't need to keep asking the same question over and over. You do need to make sure that he has a means to answer your questions. You don't need to change the location of the picture, picture symbol, or words to determine if he understands the picture, picture symbol or word.

Student #4

He is 8 years old and is known for his laugh. He has visual, physical, cognitive, and communication deficits. He is very social and delightful. At this point he is beginning to respond to yes/no questions with a head nod. He further clarifies his meaning using facial expressions.

He hasn't had consistent exposure to pictures or picture symbols at his school or home. He isn't asked questions frequently enough although he can answer my questions consistently. Increased exposure is recommended both at school and home. He has a caregiver who attends school with him. She is interested in the use of AAC and is willing to incorporate it in his daily routine at school and when she is at his home.

He has no personally prescribed communication system that meets his needs. He was provided a low-tech switch system which he has outgrown; therefore, he doesn't use it. Again, AAC systems should be ordered to include the user's need for five years. Regardless of the system ordered, five years is the standard guideline.

In addition to visuals related to the school curriculum, he has a page of symbols to address his medical needs. The use of this medical page enables him to communicate with others regarding how he is feeling and/or to inform others of his urgent medical needs. Unfortunately, it isn't used frequently.

I'm intentionally leaving out picture symbol images at this time due to licensure of software. Deciding which software to use is a book all by itself. Kids like this little guy have so much potential if those around tune into his needs and help him figure it out.

I definitely have my favorite communication systems which I share in my trainings.

AAC is Hard Work for the Student

AAC is complicated. It just is. I hear therapists instruct new AAC users saying, "You just have to do this." or "It's easy." I've been doing AAC for thirty years and it is still confusing and complex. AAC requires work initially, but the payoff is priceless.

I walked into the classroom one day and was told by the teacher "I didn't give them their devices because I didn't want them to respond." I'm certain she didn't really mean it that way. I didn't comment. Instead, I just provided the students with another means of communication while I was in the room as their devices weren't readily available.

Communicating in ways other than oral speech and using our hands for emphasis is not easy. This includes writing. I would've finished this book years ago if I just told someone and they wrote it down. I thought about it often, but I wanted to simplify this information so the material would be easier to understand.

Writing this down in a book is helping me look at the many sides and complexities of communication for those who aren't familiar with this information. I've had help from colleagues, caregivers, and friends to organize and explain this complex information. I'm truly honored by their assistance and I hope I've made my message clearer than I had it originally.

I only covered AAC briefly in my past writings because I felt there were others more qualified. One of my closest colleagues, Brad Lindner, M.S., CCC-SLP was dynamic with AAC. He was a genius! I worked with him the majority of his SLP career before he passed away suddenly in March of 2017. I miss Brad every day!

Several years prior to his death, his professional career changed from assessing and treating children who needed AAC to becoming a vendor for one of the national AAC companies. I collaborated with Brad for years in both of his roles. I soon found out that few professionals are confident within the area of AAC. One may be comfortable in one area, but not another.

I still don't call myself an AAC expert. The field changes so quickly forcing me to keep up as technology changes. Navigating the new systems, especially programming, leaves many uninterested. Those who have a system find that they can't stay within the security of having one familiar system because the hardware and software becomes outdated. Even the systems using a motor plan as its infrastructure demand us to learn the new software changes. I predominantly use one company that uses Minspeak software that doesn't change their software frequently. Fortunately, there are many therapists who are interested in keeping you afloat through these changes.

I have just a few more facts to discuss AAC. By nature, I'm a point A to point B person. AAC is not. New software is developed daily which is aimed at meeting the perfect need of the user. The only constant is that new technology has to be learned — both the hardware and software.

One challenge I compare AAC to is a corn maze. If I were to venture in one without a strategy, I would be lost forever. I learned the trick a long time ago about staying to the right side while running my hand against the right wall so I wouldn't get lost. Well, not as lost.

A similar support will lead you through the AAC maze. In AAC that support is vocabulary selection. Your client always needs vocabulary to answer yes and no questions, make a choice, and to be able to retell a story, sequence of events, and/or experience. (See Functional Communication Skills list at end of the chapter for more guidance.) Once that is established, learning and progression of the use of AAC begins!

As you probably have figured out by now my practice and my philosophy has developed and evolved over the years based on my experiences (personal and professional), my practice, and my research.

I read Helen Keller's book, *The Story of My Life* and found some eye-opening information that I thought you would like to hear too. I will link some of her thoughts with some of mine.

As I read the words penned by Helen Keller, many thoughts come to mind. I always thought Helen was born without sight and hearing; I found out that she had sight and hearing until she was about eighteen months old.

This makes a big difference when we discuss communication. She heard and she visualized within her environment for eighteen months of her life then lost it. Most likely she lost it from meningitis.

Many of the kids and adults I work with became nonverbal from various causes we discussed earlier. It is traumatic to have, then lose any sensory perception, but having the ability to see, hear, speak, and explore is a gift for communication. This gift opens doors for your ability to regain a voice to express yourself regardless of what is required for that voice. Many of my young children have this gift and then lose the ability or do not move forward with communication.

Thoughts from Helen Keller

"At the beginning, I was only a little mass of possibilities. It was my teacher who unfolded and developed them."

— Helen Keller

All nonverbal individuals need a "teacher." That "teacher" comes in many forms. It may be, you as the caregiver, therapist, or educator. No license or certification guarantees that you are the "teacher." Subsequently, not having a certification or license doesn't exclude you from being that "teacher." That is what *NOAH: The Best Gift Ever – A Voice for Everyone* is all about. This book is to help you become the "teacher" in the life of nonverbal kids and adults.

Many people, therapists as well, make the error of not giving their client enough vocabulary to develop an effective communication system. Let's take texting as an example because texting is based on vocabulary, pictures, and words. Compare the flip phone with a smartphone. A flip phone is capable of receiving/sending messages just as is a smart phone. Personally, I didn't text before the smartphone was developed; it was too cumbersome and time consuming.

Accessibility to the full keyboard made texting less challenging than having access to only nine buttons requiring me to hit the same button four times to select the letters to make words to get my message across.

AAC software was designed to provide an individual with a rich vocabulary to communicate their needs. It remains a challenge to find the best way to implement AAC, especially in the educational environment, but it can be done. The NOAH inventory was created to assist in the implementation of AAC in all environments. Some fear that the use of AAC will decrease his ability to communicate verbally.

Helen Keller has something to say about that years before technology was created.

> *"It astonished me to find how much easier*
> *it is to talk than to spell with the fingers,*
> *and I discarded the manual alphabet as*
> *a medium of communication on my part;*
> *but Miss Sullivan and a few friends still*
> *use it in speaking to me, for it is more*
> *conveniently and more rapid than lip-reading."*
>
> — Helen Keller

AAC becomes fun and even addicting once you see positive results. You will see this more in the next chapter, Habits for a Lifetime.

To conclude this chapter, I am providing a basic list of things to consider that can help guide you as you implement "THEN" and venture into the world of AAC.

The golden rule of AAC is:

"If you increase the motor demand, decrease the cognitive demand."

"If you increase the cognitive demand, decrease the motor demand."

It's easy to forget this so I typically state this multiple times in my writing and during my presentations.

Functional Communication Skills

Consider the following to develop functional communication skills using AAC:

1. Current levels of expressive, receptive, and pragmatic language. Your speech language pathologist will help you here.
2. Current cognitive functioning. I prefer a nonverbal language assessment to better meet communication needs.
3. Symbolic language usage – pictures, words, sequencing, categorization, etc.
4. Literacy skills – word prediction, letter expansion, decoding, reading comprehension, etc.
5. Motivation to use a device.
6. Support of team – individual, family, caregiver, educational support.
7. Level of physical functioning to determine access techniques such as direct select or scanning.

8. Portability – can they hold it? Does it need to be mounted to his wheelchair?
9. Switch access – what kind? Which body part or parts

A Family Affair

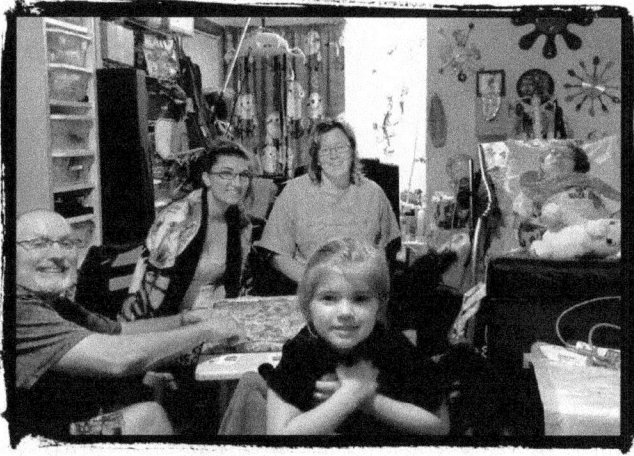

Photo courtesy of Noah's family. Edited by Paul Griesbach.

Noah's family carrying through daily activities together in his bedroom.

Chapter 8:
Habits for a Lifetime

This chapter concludes both of our mnemonics. We will focus on the "H" in NOAH and the FIND section of the mnemonic YOU CAN SEEK THEN FIND.

H stands for Habits for a Lifetime. **FIND** describes the habits that help him generalize individual skills into his conversation. This chapter is all about therapy. This chapter covers ways to make the home program fun!

NOA**H**: Habits for a Lifetime
F = Fun (YOU CAN SEEK THEN **F**IND)

Fun

Communication should be fun. Successful communication is naturally reward driven; therefore, we learn through enjoyable activities. We want something and if we communicate successfully then we usually get it. Unfortunately, fun is the component usually left out of the learning process.

NOA**H**: Habits for a Lifetime
I = Independency = (YOU CAN SEEK THEN F**I**ND)

Independent

Although communication requires a communication partner, each turn is taken independently. Keeping this in mind, independence needs to be the goal from step one. Avoid over-prompting by embedding a quick response to keep turn taking in sync. Respect the need for additional response time, while simplifying the response to preserve functional turn taking. Program his AAC device to perform this quick response. Turn taking is essential to language production.

Those who are familiar with me know that I can compare anything on Earth to the sport of soccer. AAC is no different. In soccer, independence is seen within every 1:1 opportunity. If a player cannot attain a turn when another player has the ball or maintain his turn when he already possesses the ball, he is an emerging soccer player. Another way to say that is both offensive and defensive players must be able to control the ball on their own turn with the ball and be able to take the ball away when someone else is controlling the ball.

Conversation is just like that. He needs to be able to demonstrate comprehension on his listening turn and express his needs, desires, and ideas on his expressive turn. You may already know that SLPs refer to this as pragmatic language skills. Pragmatic language skills are the social language skill components that SLPs address to promote independence in conversation.

Pragmatic language skills are lost by the age of three, if not earlier, when children are not talking. Often, I see students and adults who haven't spoken for years. The spontaneous need for a verbal turn has been lost. We interact with nonverbal kids and adults differently. Both adults and children quit interacting with those who don't respond to them.

As I'm writing in this in a coffee shop, there are two men sitting at another table nearby. My attention was drawn to them because they were making noise with their hands. I glanced over there and saw that they were exchanging turns making gestures with their hands.

Since I know sign language, I realize they are signing to each other. They are laughing and exchanging messages. Communication is independent. Both men are pulling their weight in the conversation using sign language. I chose not to interact in the conversation because I know I cannot remain independent in a sign language conversation. I can only sign with infants and toddlers!

You can retain independent turn taking by avoiding over-prompting. Embed a quick response to keep turn taking in sync whether it is a gesture, sign, picture, symbol, word, or phrase.

NOAH: Habits for a Lifetime
N = Novel (YOU CAN SEEK THEN FIND)

Novel

Communication attempts are original. Listening to a young child talking to his parents reveals originality. "Kids say the darndest things" is proof that communication is novel.

Novel means new and original. Even greetings should be novel. Think of the morning you make yourself go to work even though you should stay in bed. How many times do you lie throughout your day in response to the rote greeting "How are you?" Instead of saying "I feel horrible! I can't breathe, my throat hurts," you say, "I'm fine."

I'm realistic enough to know that rote greetings will always exist, but let's focus on teaching AAC users how to make novel expressions when we are able. Take a rote greeting and add eye contact to it. Use other pictures, picture symbols and/or words to communicate a variety of messages. Use real pictures, line drawings and videos to add variety to situations.

I've yet to find research "proving" one representation works over the other. Whatever your child, student, or loved one responds to best is the right choice. I could write a long book on all the different symbol/picture systems by itself. There are so many symbol systems because of licensure. The development of licensed symbol systems creates the need for more symbol systems. I get it. You created it so it's yours.

Licensure is important for their work, but this concept makes it difficult for the AAC user and those trying to learn how to interact with an AAC system. I have my preferences which I share in my NOAH workshops.

NOAH: Habits for a Lifetime
D = Duplicate (YOU CAN SEEK THEN FIND)

Duplicate

Language is naturally redundant for a reason. Repetition in conversation is built in subconsciously. Research shows duplication of a targeted response needs to be heard 1000 times. I don't know about you, but I hate repeating something more than twice; therefore, AAC devices, electronic toys, tablets, and other sources of technology are great to provide that duplicated response as long as it is the targeted response.

Duplication of opportunities is what creates a conversation. He must be able to activate the switch, select a picture, or imitate a word thousands of times before he communicates spontaneously. I elaborate on this in the following chapter.

Noah Loves His Cubs!

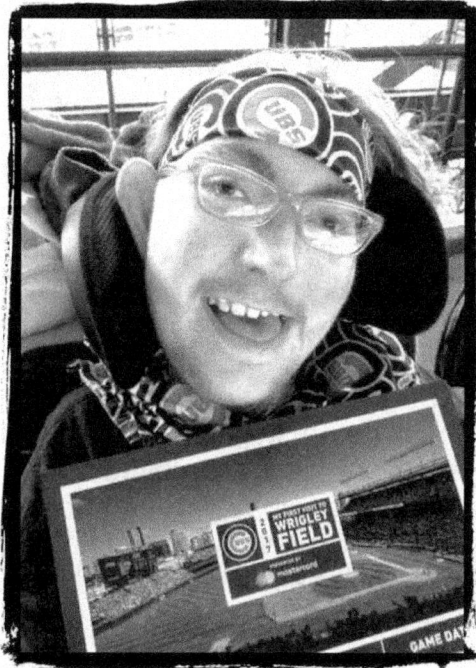

Photo courtesy of Noah's family. Edited by Paul Griesbach.

Chapter 9: Ready, Set, Go

The challenge I have in writing this book and this chapter in particular is to provide you with enough information to benefit you without turning this into a textbook or repeating too much from previous chapters. But I did promise to write this so you could read a chapter at a time when your busy routine allows so bear with me if this is repetitive for some of you.

I've tried to provide you enough of the theory and examples to illustrate the NOAH program and how to apply it through YOU CAN SEEK THEN FIND without overwhelming you. Hopefully you've already downloaded and printed the NOAH Inventory which is available on my website Lv2Pla.com so you can follow along easier. If not, this would be a good time to do so as we venture into applying it for real.

This chapter and the next three focus on one letter of NOAH and walk you through the steps of the NOAH Inventory so you can start to assess and help your loved one. If possible, try to read these four chapters close together. If you time doesn't allow, come back and review the recap below before reading each of the next three chapters.

A Quick Review

Let's get started by running through the NOAH program step by step again. If you've been reading right along and don't need this review you can skip to the next subhead (Let's Get to Work). I'm including this review because it might be helpful for some of my readers.

As you likely recall from the Introduction and Chapter 1, NOAH is an assessment and treatment program to help individuals who are nonverbal or minimally verbal that I've developed after three decades of clinical practice and have used for years with excellent results.

The mnemonic device below is based on the letters of Noah's name. Noah is a long-term client of mine who was trapped in his brain and body with little means of effective communication for years. Over and over again he and his family were told there was nothing to be done by physicians, therapists, educators — virtually everyone he encountered. His parents refused to believe that and persisted.

They now know that the real problem was that no one knew "what to do" but it came out as "there's nothing that can be done."

As you know by now if you've read the earlier chapters, my philosophy is a bit different. I view communication as a fundamental right, not a privilege. It is an ADL (Activity of Daily Living) and is essential for every living being. I don't accept "no one knows what to do" or "he can't." By assessing strengths and weaknesses and using the strengths to strengthen the weaknesses, there is always something that can be done to provide a means of communication – to give everyone a voice.

Remember NOAH stands for:

N: Nonverbal Cognitive Assessment

O: Oral Motor Intervention

A: Another Means of Communication

H: Habits for a Lifetime

The mnemonic is skills oriented for each of the four sections (or letters, if you will) of the NOAH program. As we move thorough the four Step by Step chapters (10 -13) we will focus on each one in turn.

I will simultaneously apply the mnemonic YOU CAN SEEK THEN FIND (detailed below) to teach you specific skills to address each of the sections of the NOAH program.

YOU

Y = Y̲ou do (Imitation/copying sounds and actions)
O = O̲bject Permanence (the necessary skill of knowing an object exists even when the object is out of sight)
U = U̲nderstanding (directions and questions)

CAN

C = C̲ausality – Cause-effect (action equals reaction)
A = A̲ means to an end (using available skills to get what is needed)
N = N̲eeds met (use of any communication to convey what is desired)

SEEK

S = S̲ensory (the body's response to input)
E = E̲xamine (body posture, position, and movement)
E = E̲xplore (mouth movement)
K = K̲inesiology (muscle movement)

THEN

T = T̲ogether (who he interacts with)
H = H̲ierarchy (there is an order to development)
E = E̲ngineer (create the environment)
N = N̲avigate (create successful opportunities)

FIND

F = F̲un (communication should be fun)
I = I̲ndependent (each person has a turn)
N = N̲ovel (communication is original)
D = D̲uplicate (language is naturally redundant)

Let's Get to Work

I'll teach you specific activities and strategies that you *can* do for your loved one, client or student *now*, regardless of how much or how little formal training you have. In other words, you can do some of this even if you aren't an SLP. And if you are an SLP, you can work with clients, students and families to do even more than you might have thought possible before reading about Noah and NOAH.

So let's start with the Nonverbal Cognitive Assessment. We must understand and identify his prelanguage strengths and weaknesses. If this this assessment isn't completed, I am not convinced that the evaluator truly identified his existing skills accurately.

Without identifying strengths and weaknesses, it is difficult to write goals. When we don't write intentional goals, generalization is nearly impossible.

The prelanguage skills assessment included in the nonverbal assessment is not groundbreaking, but it is new to many readers.

Since most of us can remember true words better than a collection of random letters; therefore, I use the mnemonic, "YOU CAN" to help remember the components of the nonverbal cognitive skills assessment. Let's move forward to complete a full nonverbal cognitive assessment.

Referring to the NOAH inventory will ease your ability to learn the step-by-step process of NOAH. These skills are essential for communication. In addition to the NOAH inventory and this book, I have developed products to help with the implementation of each step.

One product is "Prelanguage Priorities" which addresses the "N" of NOAH, the nonverbal cognitive assessment. I've created additional materials because a nonverbal cognitive assessment is complicated and requires further training if you aren't familiar with the components or you need to refresh your recall of these components.

I also developed a toy kit I named "Tub 'O Treasures" to help you teach him all of the early developing skills from birth to three using a plastic tub and a small number of toys/objects. I've written a manual/workbook to accompany this toy kit to establish a play routine and provide further information to get maximum benefit from these materials.

So now that we have a shared understanding and some tools to work with, let's get to work on the nonverbal cognitive assessment.

"It was my teacher's genius,

her quick sympathy,

her loving tact

which made the first

years of my education

so beautiful."

Helen Keller, *The Story of My Life* (2015)

Chapter 10: Step by Step: Nonverbal Cognitive Assessment

NOAH: Nonverbal Cognitive Assessment
Skill: Y = You Do: (YOU CAN SEEK THEN FIND)

Remember, YOU CAN SEEK THEN FIND.

YOU CAN is the step-by-step process to meet the needs of the Oral Motor Intervention of the **NOAH** program.

<u>Y</u>ou Do

Imitation is separated into three skills – gestural, vocal, and verbal. Imitation can be further divided into individual steps to make a semester long college course. We won't go there.

What it Means?

Simply put, it means to copy. Copy a facial expression, copy a movement, copy a sound, copy a word, or copy a sentence. In order to copy, he has to be able to sustain attention long enough to figure out what to copy. Next, he has to figure out how to carry out the motor part of the plan to copy. Finally, he successfully copies or imitates the facial expression, the gesture, the sound, or the word.

How to Assess?

Regardless of age, keep it simple. Use your eyes and your ears. Smile, does he imitate you? Smiling is contagious. If he imitates your smile, show him a few facial expressions such as an exaggerated eye opening, scrunch your nose, stick-out your tongue, etc. Now mark your score sheet with (+) or (-). Yes, it is difficult to assess if he possesses severe motor deficits but not impossible. Just figure out which muscles he can control. Begin with his eye muscles.

Move onto gestures and body movements. Give him a high five, fist bump, clap hands, or wave. This shows us his ability to respond to a natural movement and to copy. Signing is a verbal communication skill. It is an alternate verbal skill not included in gesture imitation. Imitation of words is the most advanced form of imitation.

What If He Can't Imitate?

It is fair to say that he who can't talk, can't imitate yet. There are few exceptions. Failure to imitate is not always due to cognitive or language reasons; it may be due to a motor impairment – weakness (dysarthria) or motor sequence (apraxia). We'll discuss that further as we explore ways to develop imitation and oral motor intervention.

Your responsiveness to their imitation is important to increase the likelihood they will imitate you again. If his attempts aren't reinforced, soon he will stop imitating. I see this often. Imitation is present but not demonstrated because the behavior was actually extinguished by not responding to the behavior. For example, when he raises his hands up to communicate "pick me up," he will repeat this nonverbal communication attempt if you respond to his request by actually picking him up. If he isn't responded to when he uses the gesture to be picked up, he will stop raising his hands to communicate this intention.

Ways to Develop Imitation

Imitation is a complex skill. This is usually the last of the prelanguage cognitive skills to develop. There are many things to do that encourage imitation development.

Although development of this skill is complex, don't make it more complicated. The medical and educational communities make it way too hard.

Play is the answer. Make silly faces to your loved one. Act like his favorite character or dance to his favorite song. For adults, help him relive his memories/experiences. Sing the old commercial jingles with adults. "I am stuck on Band-Aid", "Have it Your Way," "Two all-beef patties, special sauce…"

95

Whatever works — a funny face, a high-five, a fist bump, a random gesture — do it! Do it again and again. Make it a game for him to copy. Imitation will come. Length of time varies, but it will come in lightbulb fashion.

What do I mean? You will know when imitation of facial expressions, body movements, sounds, and words occur, and it looks like the skill happened out of the blue just as the light bulb illuminates when an unseen person flips the switch. It will just suddenly happen if you keep at it.

Imitation of pointing to pictures or touching a touch screen or activating a voice output device is another form of communication. Your job is to increase the number of opportunities.

Remember we are working on non-verbal imitation: expression, motor movements and gestures which will eventually lead to the highest form of imitation — words. Imitation of words may be difficult to see at first. He may imitate you in a way that sounds like random strings of consonant-vowel combinations that SLPs call babbling. He may also imitate words perfectly clear, but this is rare.

Functional Activities within Daily Routines

A functional activity is simply something he needs to do today. An infant must be able to suck to get food, bat a toy to make it play music, or respond to an adult's facial expression. Functional activities for adults include rotary tongue movement to swallow food, activating a remote control, swiping a tablet, waving to greet someone, and nodding their head to indicate yes or no.

Singing songs with hand movements is a great way to develop imitation skills. Reading a book to them with simplified language also promotes participation; therefore, imitation. Simplified language could mean the use of pictures, AAC symbols, or other visual strategies. I've included pictures in our "Little Paul" series to allow your loved one or clients to retell the story. You will need the help of therapists to fully create pictures, symbols for his daily routines.

NOAH: Nonverbal Cognitive Assessment
Skill: O = Object Permanence: (YOU CAN SEEK THEN FIND)

<u>O</u>bject Permanence
What it Means

Object permanence is the prelanguage skill prerequisite to labeling or naming objects and people. Object permanence is knowing an object exists even when you can't see it.

How to Assess?

There are different levels of object permanence. Initial development in infancy is to cry when mom leaves the room. Soon after, it's finding a toy that is hidden by something such as a blanket. The level increases by the complexity of the hidden object. For example, the toy is hidden under a blanket then under another object then into a closed hand. Finally, he can climb on top of the kitchen counter to get on the shelf to get the cookies from the cookie jar.

Assessing object permanence if he has limited hand movement is a bit tougher. Does he move his eyes to follow the object? I frequently see him look at the object; he follows it to the next hiding spot and so forth. Hand use is not required to demonstrate object permanence. Another way of saying that is he can learn the cognitive skill of object permanence even if he can't use his hands. We have to make sure we give him opportunities to learn object permanence in his own way. We have to observe to see how he is demonstrating object permanence. Yes, identifying his own "way" may take time.

On the NOAH inventory I write "follows until object disappears" which means simply that. If he follows the object until it's out of sight, the basic level of object permanence is present. If

97

He cannot follow the object until it is out of sight, he has not achieved the first level of object permanence yet.

"One screen" means if I cover it so the object is hidden. He can find it.

"Two screens" means I can hide the object in one location then another. He will be able to know you are hiding the object for a second time and can find it. I use a blanket or a covered box to play this hiding game.

"Three screens" means I can take an object from him (such as my keys) and put them in my hand. As I close my hand, I put them in my purse. Afterwards, I move my purse to the table. If he can let me know the keys are in the purse, he has achieved the level of three screens. Once he achieves this level there is only one more level to achieve.

This final level is when he can find anything (such as a cookie in a closed cookie jar) even when it is hidden in something that that does not all ow him to see inside. This level makes it truly impossible to hide anything from him.

What If He Can't?

If you aren't yet aware that an object is present when you can't see the object, you won't need a word to request the object. If I see the object, I can grab it. If I don't see the object, I have forgotten about the object and do not know that I want it; therefore, the need for a word isn't necessary. Until this skill develops, words aren't necessary. We want to help him develop this skill as soon as possible.

Ways to Develop Object Permanence

Children can play with you if you hide toys/objects. Hidden can mean partially hidden with an edge of the object showing. Find out what toy he prefers, then hide it under one object such as a blanket or scarf. Hide the object in a box with a lid. My favorite toys for developing this skill are the toys that fall down to the bottom of the toy box such as fast-food kids' meal toys or their favorite TV show characters. Work on the use of eye gaze doing the same thing. Let him find the object using his eyes. Object permanence is seen in adults by finding the remote for the tv, their medic alert remote, their cell phone or other electronics. Knowing that there is a bottle of water in their refrigerator or pills in their pill box.

Make sure you are accommodating for visual, hearing, and/or motor impairments. You will need therapists input for these accommodations.

Functional Activities within Daily Routines

He can play with toys such as blocks, animals, or cars as you create the hiding spots. You may also use food such as cereal or gummy bears and hide it in containers. When assessing an adult, he may indicate object awareness or function by gesturing its use or pointing in the general direction. You can work on these skills throughout their daily routines.

NOAH: Nonverbal Cognitive Assessment
Skill: U = Understand Directions, Commands
(YO<u>U</u> CAN SEEK THEN FIND)

<u>U</u>nderstand
What it Means?

In order to carry on a conversation, he must be able to understand what is being said. Sustained attention is a prerequisite to understanding what is being said to him Sustained attention refers to how long he attends to a person, activity, or object. Being instructed in his language such as picture symbols, enhanced visuals that reflect light, or using something such as a light box or electronic tablet is essential for an AAC user. Can he understand directions? Can he follow directions?

How to Assess?

No formal test is required to figure out his ability to follow commands or respond to questions. Give a few commands to determine comprehension. You might tell a child to do something with an object (i.e. put it in the box, kiss Elmo, or tickle Daddy). You can ask an adult to put the pen on the paper, point to the ceiling, or clap his hands). Ask him yes and no questions. The ability to respond to yes and no questions using a body part increases your loved one's ability to engage in conversation. *I can't emphasize that enough.*

Of course, these directions must be attainable for the person. He must be able to perform the task. If he can't use his hands, say something such as "look at Mommy," look at the door," "open your mouth," etc. Have fun with this! He is more likely to show he has the ability to follow directions and respond to questions if he is easily engaged in the activity. Look for those nonverbal ways he is communicating to you. Can he understand the 5 w's and h questions? Who, what, when, where, why and how?

The NOAH inventory checklist also assesses his hearing response by including response to auditory stimuli such as a startle and localizing. Localizing simply means he can identify where the sound came from and turns his head towards that location. Hearing screenings and assessment is imperative for children and adults to ensure that he hears all frequencies of sound.

What If He Can't?

Before kids learn to answer questions and follow directions, we have different expectations. Babies are very young, under the age of one, when they respond to their name, "want up?," "where's mommy?" or "give me."

If he can't follow directions or answer questions, you need to start asking questions and providing simple directions to follow such as those listed above. Keep it simple. Play with him and look for the way he interacts with you. You may be missing the nonverbal communication he is using to answer your question or respond to your direction. Have the expectation that he *will* answer your questions and follow your directions.

Develop Understanding of Directions and Questions

There is a natural hierarchy to questioning response with yes or no questions being first and w questions (what, who, where, when, why, and how) developing later. With that being said, people don't read the language manual and do not necessarily develop these skills in sequential order.

Yes or no question response is always a goal for me because it opens up a line of communication in form and range of intention. Worth repeating again, yes or no responses should be developed using a body part if at all possible, such as a head nod. When using symbols, I choose the yes or no symbols that shows a child nodding his head to direct to the use of a body part to indicate yes or no. Always work toward a motor response using his body so his yes or no answer is easily communicated to others.

Functional Activities within Daily Routines

For children: "Do you want a cookie?" "Do you want to take a nap?", "Put it in the trash," and "Sit down" are the first commands we tend to use. Much later you will see the development of questions and directives such as "After you finish your supper, you may have dessert."

This still works for me.

For adults we ask: "What show do you want to watch?", " What's your name?", "What day is it?", "Where are you?" or we say "stick out your tongue", "swallow again," "match the word to the picture," "do ten leg lifts or count to ten", etc.

101

<u>N</u>OAH: Nonverbal Cognitive Assessment
Skill: C = Causality (YOU <u>C</u>AN SEEK THEN FIND)

<u>C</u>ausality
What it Means?

Causality simply means having the ability to cause an effect. You know your child is demonstrating causality when he throws the keys on the floor for the fifth time knowing you will pick them up. I frequently see kids hitting switches repetitively. This may or may not indicate awareness of causality. Causality is when they know something is going to happen.

The NOAH inventory includes the following items to mark off. Does he examine his own hands? Can he reactivate a toy previously activated? Does he try to use an adult's hand to reactivate the toy? Does he observe the action of the toy moving? Finally, can he turn the object on/off or reactivate the toy independently? This skill includes turning on a musical toy, a phone, remote control, tablet, medical alert device or hearing aid.

How to Assess?

This skill is assessed by observing a child in play or an adult carrying out their daily routines. For a child, causality progresses from batting a toy and making it move independently to activating a toy to make it play more music, spin, or other function. For an adult, causality is demonstrated through controlling the TV with a remote, activating a medical alert button after falling, setting a timer, or playing a game on a mobile phone, electronic tablet, or computer.

What If He Can't?

Causality is an essential skill for the development of communication. If he can't cause an effect, he can't play with a toy for very long because the play ends. This is true for a child playing with Elmo or an adult playing Solitaire on a tablet. He can't make another person interact with him or request assistance from another.

102

For adults, this may also include turning on his hearing aid, activating an electric can opener, or turning on music. We need this skill in order to communicate.

Ways to Develop Causality

The nonverbal aspects of causality are essential to cognitive functioning and the development of communication skills regardless of age. You can have him learn this through toy play. He needs to know how to use an adult to activate a toy he is unable to activate or how to push a button to make an electronic toy work. He discovers how objects work using this skill. Adults need to know how to activate electronic devices such as the phone, computer, or a TV through repetition of these controls. He will use these skills to interact with others. He needs these skills to activate any form of augmentative/alternative communication (AAC).

Functional Activities within Daily Routines

Children need to know how to play with toys, objects, and the people around them. Adults need to know how to interact with people and use objects around them such as phones, microwave ovens, TV remotes, tablets, computers, and medial alert devices to assist in their medical care and/or needs with caregivers.

NOAH: Nonverbal Cognitive Assessment
Skill: A = A means end (YOU C<u>A</u>N SEEK THEN FIND)
<u>A</u> Means End

What it Means?

Means end simply refers to figuring out how to get your hands (or controlling another's) to get what you want. Problem solving is another way of describing means end. Means end looks quite different for kids and adults with minimal use of their hands. The first area to look at is how they can access an object without being able to grab the object. Means end drives the ability to use other skills to get what we want. It is essential to comprehend how to assess to move your client forward.

How to Assess?

I look at his facial expressions, eye gaze, head turn and other body language. Instead of having him place his hands on

103

a string on the toy to pull it off the table, we have to look at how he communicates with us to pull the object off of the table for him. It comes with practice. Mark down your findings on the NOAH inventory.

What If He Can't?

Addressing the absence of means end is more difficult to explain because it's a higher-level cognitive skill which needs to be present for communication intention to develop.

Following the checklist on the NOAH inventory, he needs to be able to move an object to get another, pull the support such as a blanket under the toy he can't quite reach, or communicate to his caregiver that he wants that desired object. Once means end is present, he will get into everything or indicate what he desires. Means end is the skill that motivates the toddler to crawl, cruise, and walk because he has the desire to get something.

Working with other therapists and educators, it is my job to facilitate the development of cognitive skills to help him develop motor skills. In the nonverbal community, this means I work on developing the prelanguage cognitive skills to develop motor planning. The use of AAC, even the lowest tech available, helps him develop prelanguage skills to develop a communication system.

As you can imagine, means end is a tough skill for kids and adults with motor deficits to learn. It just means we have to target these skills and work on them daily. You may want to explore products on my website Lv2Pla.com for resources to help you and your loved one or client on your journey.

Ways to Develop Means End

This skill is developed by providing time for him to problem solve regardless of age. Time for problem solving is essential. Add cues to help but not take over the problem solving. Watch him as he tries to get the desired object off the table or to change the channel on the remote. Give him time to activate a switch with his hands, eyes, feet, toes, etc. Help him explore to achieve whatever it takes to get his message across. Mark your findings on the NOAH inventory.

Functional Activities within Daily Routines

The major difference between causality and means end is the problem-solving factor. He has to figure out how to accomplish his goal. Functional activities are simply those activities he wants to accomplish. It's an early form of goal setting. He wants the book he can't reach requiring assistance. This assistance may come in the form of pointing, gesturing, climbing on the table, countertop, etc. It may also come in the form of activating an AAC device with his fingers, head, or toes, or eyes to tell someone else how to make the movement occur.

NOAH: Nonverbal Cognitive Assessment
Skill: N = Needs met (YOU CA<u>N</u> SEEK THEN FIND)
<u>N</u>eeds Met

What it Means?

It simply means the use of nonverbal and verbal communication to get what you need. Needs are met through the combination of nonverbal and verbal communication. We will look at communication intentions categorized by the range of intentions and the form of intentions. Range of intention is categorized as requests, comments, labels, protests, and questions. Form of intention is categorized as reflexive sounds, crying, babbling, use of gestures, facial expressions, words, signs, etc.

How to Assess?

Following the NOAH inventory checklist, mark off how he is able to have his needs met. Does he cry? Does he whine or make other nonverbal noise with purpose to express himself? Is he able to point to what he wants to make a request? Is he able to say a word or use an AAC system?

What If He Can't?

The first step is observation. It is rare that he isn't trying to communicate using one of the forms I listed above. The next step is, completing the remainder of the NOAH inventory to develop a strategy.

Ways to Develop Needs Met

Observation is key to understanding needs met. Listen to his cry, his babble, and his word approximations. Look at his facial expressions, his gestures, his sign and/or word approximations. This is true for children and adults. Humans are always trying to communicate despite exhibiting multiple deficits.

Functional Activities to Develop Needs Met

Children make requests, a nice word for demands, from infancy. Around the age of 10 months, he begins making these requests with purpose. We call that intentional communication.

From that stage of development and forward, the focus should be on increasing his range of these intentions and his form of intentions. Requesting the desired cookie by eye gaze then crying, then vocalizing to signs and/or use of words. There is a general hierarchy of development. Rarely will someone learn a word then go back to crying without some form of neurological or behavioral change. Like the quote I shared earlier from Helen Keller, "It astonished me to find how much easier it is to talk than to spell with fingers, and I discarded the manual alphabet as a medium of communication on my part." Finding a means to communicate is essential if you want him to communicate his needs. Finding that means of communication now is the expectation. Don't wait!

This completes the **YOU CAN,** the nonverbal cognitive assessment of the NOAH inventory. Now we will continue with SEEK THEN FIND to add oral intervention for speech and provide him with another means to communicate.

It's Not What It Looks Like

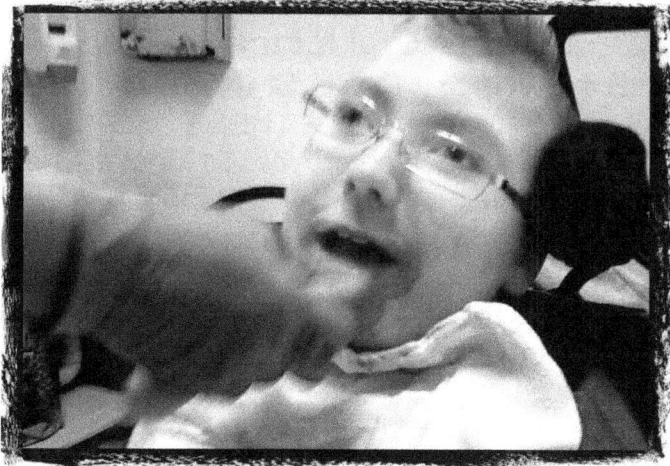

Photo courtesy of Noah's family. Edited by Paul Griesbach.

**No need for concern. Really. It's cherry juice.
However, Laura did a doubletake when
Noah's Dad posted this picture on Facebook.**

Chapter 11: Step by Step: Oral Motor Intervention

N<u>O</u>AH: Oral Motor Invention
Skill: S = Sensory (YOU CAN <u>S</u>EEK THEN FIND)

Remember, YOU CAN SEEK THEN FIND.

SEEK is the step-by-step process to meet the needs of the Oral Motor Intervention of the **NOAH** program.

<u>Sensory</u>
What It Means

Sensory refers to the body's response to tactile, auditory, visual, smell, taste, proprioception, and vestibular stimuli. Sensory assessment will facilitate tolerance if hypersensitive and/or increase arousal if hyposensitive in response to stimuli. To simplify this thought, it is important to know how his body responds to stimulation. If he responds more than what is expected or not enough, we will need to work on normalizing his response.

Personally, I don't meet anyone for the first time and stick one of those pink or green swabs in his mouth and establish hyper/normal/hypo response. I establish rapport with him and may not even touch his mouth at all that day. Sensory processing is another one of "those" areas so many want to debate. Avoiding wasting time on that debate, you will be able to see progress quicker. Adequate sensory processing is imperative for attention skills. Sustained attention is imperative for learning. Traditionally, occupational therapists perform the comprehensive sensory processing assessment and write a report.

How to Assess?

We need to assess all areas of sensory input. A team approach, as I describe below, is best.

Auditory

You either have a formal report or you are screening his hearing. All of our kids and adults need to have a formal hearing test if he fails a screening. If at all possible, he needs a formal hearing test from an audiologist.

Visual

You either have a formal report or you are screening his vision. If at all possible, he needs a formal vision assessment from a vision specialist. Neuro-ophthalmologists and low vision specialists are two of the best-kept secrets in the field. Don't hesitate to refer. Therapists should attend the appointment if at all possible. You can help him communicate and address your specific concerns with the specialist.

Proprioceptive

Traditionally occupational therapists assess this area when we are looking at sensory processing. It is defined as reacting to stimuli that are produced and perceived within oneself, especially those connected with the position and movement of one's body. This concept is so important for all kids and adults. It helps him figure out where he is in space and how to plan out motor movements.

Tactile

This relates to the sense of touch. Most frequently we are talking about touching with his hands or his body being passively touched. It also includes exploring with his mouth. You may be familiar with the expressions tactile sensitive, tactile aversion, and tactile defensive. These terms are commonly used to qualify if the tactile system is functional. SLPs, PTs, and OTs evaluate different parts of the body to determine if tactile skills are within normal functional limits.

Vestibular

This relates to the inner ear and his sense of balance. PTs and OTs are your "go to" for assessment of vestibular skills. This is an important area of SEEK because the sense of balance relates to his ability to tolerate movement as well as improving balance or maintaining balance. There is decreased overall movement in our kids and adults restrained in their wheelchair for long periods of time.

Does he have a prior diagnosis of sensory processing disorder? This may also be referred to as sensory integration disorder. If this is already documented, find out if he is receiving therapy for this or if there are accommodations are in place.

I said traditionally OTs complete this assessment, but other therapists and educators are trained in this as well. That being said, I refer to OT or other trained therapist for a full sensory processing assessment. Utilizing each discipline's strengths improves his functional performance. This allows the SLP to focus on oral motor skills under SEEK.

Keeping practicality in mind, my goal is to provide you with information to realize the importance of oral motor intervention. I am excited to say that many colleagues now see the importance of oral intervention in speech development.

Let's get started. Assessment begins with positioning. Whether positioned in a chair or wheelchair, oral skills are captured best in the seated position. An example of skills check-off:

Trunk control	(+) or (-)	Max support required
Body Ground	(+) or (-)	Max support required

Mark your findings on the NOAH inventory.

In order for appropriate oral development, head and trunk control must be present. Professionals tend to get preoccupied with the concept of midline. I choose to focus on the body being grounded. Firm support beneath us, whether feet or seat, is the input required to help us know where our body is in space. Grounding of our body helps us tolerate the input from our senses. To ensure adequate grounding, have him sit down. When sitting he needs to have his anatomical seat in the seated position. The lower back is naturally supported in a chair with a seat back and adaptively supported in a wheelchair. This sounds simple, but this is the number one failure when seated.

Now that he is seated properly let's see how the feet are grounded. Frequently, his feet are swinging under his seat or sticking out in front. Have him put his feet on the floor or on the footrest. Don't be afraid to use the straps to hold his feet on the footrest.

Now that he is sitting appropriately it's time to look how his arms are positioned. Don't get caught up on his ability or inability to use his arms. Don't worry about etiquette. He needs his arms resting on something – arms of chair, the tabletop, the tray top, etc. Our arms go somewhere even if they rest on our lap. Do his arms rest on the table? His lap? the armrest? Or do his arms spread outward, behind his back, or in ATNR (asymmetrical tonic neck reflex).

Although I don't get caught up on the concept of midline, I do facilitate arms maintained near midline. When positioned in the sitting position, he tends to leave his nondominant arm in a non-functioning position. If he exhibits ATNR he needs additional support to prevent his arms from falling behind him. It takes too much energy for him to bring his arms back into the midline position.

For adults, the struggle may be having residual weakness or paralysis from a stroke. Head support is crucial in the sitting position as well. This is the number one thing I struggle with when addressing feeding. If he is sitting in his wheelchair without a tray, he may have difficulty reaching the table. Please address this in a manner other than an awkward position at a table. Adaptations to allow for arm stabilization is required. Tables of varying height helps with positioning, especially when you have many clients in wheelchairs of varying heights.

Now that he is sitting with adequate head and trunk control in combination with a grounded body position, he is ready to work.

What If He Can't

Any signs of sensory deficits need to be addressed. Therapy and accommodations are recommended to allow him to process all sensory information. His strengths and weaknesses need to be documented so we can help him progress in the weak areas or note a deficit such as blindness or deafness. Goals in these areas are essential. Many AAC software programs rely on motor planning which relies on sensory input.

Oral motor sensory deficits are a red flag for a swallowing disorder and/or speech production.

Ways to Develop

I just said that we need to improve sensory input response to as close as normal as possible. Physical, occupational, and speech therapy will address these deficits in therapy. They will help you develop a treatment plan and a home exercise plan.

Functional Activities

I especially want to keep this area short because the activities vary by his areas of strengths and weaknesses. Some common interventions are deep pressure, heavy work, oral massage, calming, and increased exposure to stimuli that bothers them. There are so many fun activities that can easily be incorporated in his activities of daily living.

N<u>O</u>AH: Oral Motor Invention
Skill: E = <u>E</u>xamine (YOU CAN S<u>E</u>EK THEN FIND)

<u>E</u>xamine
What it Means?

It is important to examine his whole-body posture and his position. By understanding how his body is moving, we will be able to understand how his mouth is moving in desired and undesired ways. How is his head control? Does he have adequate head control? What support does he require?

How to Assess?

Look at his ability to move his muscles. Frequently, I work with kids and adults who have extremely limited use of their hands. We're looking at his ability to use his mouth muscles. On occasion I limit the use of a specific muscles or groups of muscles to encourage the use of different muscles or groups of muscles.

For example, I may place his arms in the armrests of his chair then Velcro the armrest attachments to position his arms fully in the arm rests. This decreases reflexive movement I don't want to elicit. With his arm movement restricted, he is able to control his head, face, neck, and mouth muscles easier. It is easier to control one area of muscles than all the muscles in the body simultaneously.

Follow the NOAH inventory "Examine" portion. Look for symmetry of appearance and strength of the lips, tongue, smile, and jaw position. Mark (+) or (-) accordingly on the NOAH Inventory.

What If He Can't?

This section is easy to mark presence or absence and note whether his mouth structures are symmetrical in appearance and strength. Look at his smile, jot down anything that looks different about his smile. This may seem unimportant, but this can make the difference in having the ability to eat by mouth and speak clearly.

It is nearly impossible to have adequate jaw stability, strength, and coordination if symmetrical alignment isn't present. If he is unable to move his tongue side to side, it negatively impacts his ability to reach the surfaces that his tongue must come in contact with to produce n, t, d, s, l, r, z, sh, ch, and /jz/ like in jar.

This isn't a strength issue but a movement issue. No one questions that it is difficult to use his fingers if he is unable to open his hand. This is the idea. If his tongue can't reach the top of his mouth, the lower part of his mouth by his top and bottom teeth, or various positions which require him to hold his tongue there long enough for the sound to be produced such as r, sh, ch, and jz as in jar his speech will not be clear.

I'm trying to keep this simple enough to understand but reveal the complexities of speech production at the same time.

Look at his smile, jot down anything that looks different about his smile on your copy of the NOAH Inventory.

Ways to Develop

Now you're looking at your copy of the NOAH inventory and what you wrote down. Simple exercises have been created for the mouth just as there are simple exercises for weak leg muscles. Muscles are muscles; they change when we use them. You don't have to know all the ins and outs about muscle development to appreciate if I sit on the couch all winter, my muscles will be weak come springtime.

Functional Daily Activities

The easiest way to keep your mouth muscles strong is to eat and talk. These are the two things most commonly impacted if he cannot speak and has difficulty swallowing.

I was surprised to see this sentence in Helen Keller's book I referred to earlier: "My friends say that I laughed and cried naturally, and for a while I made many sounds and word elements, not because they were a means of communication, but because the need of exercising my vocal organs was imperative."

We now know that many vocalizations and what some refer to as grunting are word approximations. Word approximations are his attempts to say words, but these words are unintelligible or difficult to understand. When we sort out the pattern of consonant productions, we find out he is saying words.

Vocalizations are simply speech attempts when the tongue, lips, and teeth aren't used in a way that produces consonant sounds. A fairly easy way to differentiate between verbalizations and vocalizations is the presence of consonant sound in verbalizations and the absence of consonant sounds in vocalizations.

Those that know me, hear me frequently say "all we need are consonant sounds combined with vowels to give him credit for that vocal attempt to become a word." Then it only takes words strung together to make him a verbal communicator.

The most important thing you can do to help the nonverbal child or adult in your life is to talk to him and expect him to respond. Try to get him to repeat what you think he is saying or what would be the most likely verbal comment he would be saying during that opportunity by speaking those words for him.

NOAH: Oral Motor Invention
Skill: E =Explore (YOU CAN SEEK THEN FIND)

Explore
What it Means?

While the "Examine" portion of the NOAH inventory is for you to perform as the examiner, the "Explore" portion of NOAH inventory is what he must do by himself.

We are looking to see how much he is able to explore mouth movements using the primary articulators. Articulators is the fancy word to describe when the surfaces of the lips, tongue, teeth, jaws, and/or palate touch or articulate each other. These movements tell us why he is able to say certain sounds and/or why he is unable to say consonant sounds at all. It also provides us with information about his ability to eat and drink.

This area is complicated when swallowing skills are of concern. Referring to a speech-language pathologist for a complete swallowing assessment is your first step if he manages his saliva by drooling or he requires suctioning.

How to Assess?

This section describes what he needs to do versus you doing it for him. As I mentioned earlier, little boys show us a great model for sound exploration. Typically, speech and language development is slower for boys, but sound exploration comes early for boys. Little boys make sounds when imagining that a stick is a sword, microphone, or animal.

We need to help in a passive manner so he can move his tongue, lips, and facial muscles to produce a sound. Watch a little boy's mouth when he is playing. You will see constant motion. This step of the process develops through spontaneous exploration. Follow along the NOAH inventory with me please and we will master this section together.

We are looking to see if he can move his tongue independently. Is he able to explore the inside of his cheeks, the back molar region of his mouth, and the complete top portion of his mouth which includes the soft and hard palates? Is he able to stick his tongue out of his mouth without the support of the lips? This is referred to as tongue protrusion.

Who ever thought it would be important to stick your tongue out at someone? This isn't so much a strength issue as one of range of motion. Our tongue muscles are amazingly complicated. The tongue is made up of many muscles connected together. Although I'm breaking this down into just a few muscle movements and trying to simplify the process, you can make a difference in his life working on these simple movements. Now circle all the consonant sounds he can say on the NOAH inventory. That's it for our assessment.

Ways to Develop

Earlier I talked about ways to develop the mouth muscles. Remember this section is how he explores his mouth independently. However, passive oral exercises may be the place to begin. Passive exercises are the movements we do for him until he can do them himself.

Being the overachiever that I am, I had a knee replacement at the age of 47. My awesome physical therapist started me with passive leg exercises until I developed enough strength to do the same exercises independently. Doing those passive exercises *worked*! Don't think for a moment that passive means useless movement. I am thankful for my PT who worked with me until I learned to walk again! Passive exercising has its role in muscle development.

We will talk more about muscle change in the next section, Kinesiology.

N<u>O</u>AH: Oral Motor Invention
Skill: K = <u>K</u>inesiology (YOU CAN SEE<u>K</u> THEN FIND)

<u>K</u>inesiology
What it Means?

This is a fancy word for the study of the way muscles are moving. We can change muscle movements by knowing how the muscles work together.

Yes, you are right. This one is a bit more confusing, but don't put the book down quite yet. I will explain this in a way you can get right to work on making improvements.

This step completes the oral motor intervention section. I want to increase his awareness of his body. Oral motor responds to stimulation; therefore, we need to stimulate his muscles to increase his awareness of these muscles.

Consonant production is dependent on oral movements by which we make two or more surfaces of the mouth touch each other. Vowel production does not require the same amount of work or detail. Although we are unable to change the reason causing the delay in muscle development, we are able to change the impact to the muscles using kinesiology facts. We are able to change the muscle fibers in the mouth just as we do any other muscle in the human body.

How to Assess?

This area of the NOAH program is also very simplified. I will not make you a kinesiologist, but my hope is to increase your awareness of muscle development. The assessment for this portion of the NOAH inventory was completed in the sensory, examine, and explore portions.

The final question you have to ask yourself is simple. Can he move his oral muscles independently (active muscle movement) or does he need your help to move his oral muscles (passive muscle movement)?

What If He Can't?

If he requires a passive oral exercise program, that is where we begin. If he requires an active oral exercise program, that is where we begin. Don't be discouraged if he requires a passive oral exercise program. That's where I usually begin.

Ways to Develop

Now that you have reached this portion of the NOAH inventory, please turn back to Chapter 5 and thoroughly read the Oral Motor intervention section if you have not already done so or if it's been a while since you read that chapter.

A referral to a speech-language pathologist for a complete speech and swallowing assessment is highly recommended. They will help you develop a home program individualized for your loved one. If you are an SLP reading this and saying I know little about oral motor intervention and/or swallowing there are many courses available on those topics. With a little training, you will be an expert to help all those in need who live around you.

Beach Bound

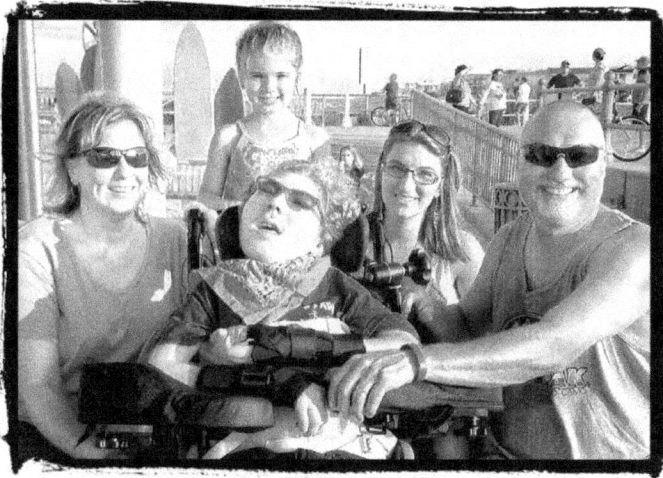

Photo courtesy of Noah's family. Edited by Paul Griesbach.

Noah's AAC is part of his life no matter where he and his family go.

Chapter 12: Step by Step: Another Means to Communicate
NOAH:　Another Means to Communicate
Skill:　T = Together (YOU CAN SEEK THEN FIND)

Remember, YOU CAN SEEK THEN FIND.

THEN is the step-by-step process to meet the needs of the Another Means to Communicate portion of the NOAH program.

Together
What It Means

Together answers the question "Who does he interact with?"

Following along with your copy of the NOAH inventory you will see multiple lines to complete a comprehensive list of who he interacts with. Too often those who are unable to speak, communicate with their parents, caregivers, teachers and medical personnel only. We can help him tremendously by increasing the number and variety of people he interacts with. This is another area where Noah's family excels!

How to Assess?

You can simply complete the lines provided for you on the NOAH inventory to summarize who he interacts with throughout his day. I referred to the *Social Networks: A Communication Inventory for Individuals with Complex Communication Needs and their Communication Partners* by Sara W. Blackstone, Ph. D. and Mary Hunt Berg, Ph.D. earlier in the book. I find this inventory helpful to teach others how to increase the number and variety of social interactions for my nonverbal kids and adults.

What If He Can't?

Simply put, increase the number of people and the variety of interactions he can participate in. He is dependent on the opportunities we make available for him. This will help you too. Both client and caregiver need a support system in place.

Ways to Develop

Encourage participation with others at home, in school, church, clubs, support groups, etc. Think outside of the box. I've observed my clients' families and am in awe at the opportunities they find or create.

Many of the kids I've worked with experience family vacations, community experiences such as attending ball games or playing on a team. They create play dates that continue to amaze me. To complete this assessment, it may be starting with adding just one more person for your kid to interact with such as a neighbor or a grandparent.

Another area of importance is communication with medical providers whether it's to schedule an appointment with his doctor or to text his therapist of a wonderful moment, both client and caregiver should be able to add this form of communication to his daily life.

H = Hierarchy (YOU CAN SEEK THEN FIND)
Hierarchy
What it Means?

For the development of most things in life there is a hierarchy or an order to how things develop. I've included the order of Augmentative and Alternative Communication (AAC) development in the NOAH Program.

AAC is most commonly described in three levels: Emerging, Context Dependent, and Independent.

The first level, the *emerging communicator,* is just beginning to explore AAC.

The *context dependent communicator* is best described as the second level of AAC communication. He is dependent on others to help him use AAC. He requires others to set up his opportunities to communicate. He knows how to hit a switch but isn't able to independently access the vocabulary. He is just learning that he can request help. He still needs others to show him with whom he should be communicating and what AAC to use. At this stage, he is still finding where the messages he desires to say are located, when to use AAC, why he needs to communicate and how to use his AAC system(s).

The final level is the *independent* AAC user. This is exactly what it says. An independent user can do whatever he needs to do with his device(s) to communicate. He will still need assistance to support his motor deficits such as setting up the device up, programming the device, troubleshooting, or other technical supports which don't count against independence.

How to Assess?

Observation is the best way to assess this area. This is the easiest area to assess on the whole NOAH inventory! Is he able to use his AAC device(s) independently, does he need help to use his device, or is he just beginning his use of AAC? Keep in mind that we are looking at his ability to communicate. We are looking at functional communication skills. We don't teach how to use the device, but how to communicate using the device.

What If He Can't?

There is no can't.

I always begin at the level where he and his caregiver are currently. To be honest with you, through the past 30 years, I have only had a handful of individuals become an independent AAC user. Why is this? I believe the reason for this is because individuals who cannot speak do not receive therapy, education, social opportunities, or even medical care the same way those who can speak. Adding AAC intervention when the child is four is much easier to make happen than at the age of 25 or 75.

Ways to Develop

I have worked with individuals ranging from premature infants born at 25 weeks gestation to adults 103 year of age who are unable to express themselves and have a few stories to share about their progress from receiving services early.

I think we are making progress in a program where I'm currently providing speech therapy and assistive technology. The problem is this is just one small area. Training families, therapists, educators, physicians, nurses, case managers, and the list goes on is key.

Early referral and identification are the answer to moving kids and adults through this hierarchy to develop independent AAC use. In fact, this is the whole point of this book. I'm writing to increase awareness of the number of individuals who remain "trapped in" for a lifetime because no one knows what to do.

After reading this book and completing the NOAH Inventory and related activities you won't have to accept that "no one knows what to do" because now, *you* do. You can advocate for and help your loved one or client or student because you know.

Yes, now you do!

E = Engineer (YOU CAN SEEK TH<u>E</u>N FIND)
Engineer
What it Means?

It is essential to create an environment to make communication happen. We have to anticipate his communication needs and make it happen.

Earlier. I mentioned that the use of AAC is not a natural process. That being said we need to make it more natural and teach how to move through the levels we just discussed: emerging, context dependent, and independent.

From the time we present AAC to him, we need to be working on decreasing our assistance to help him use the device independently. Another way of saying this is to engineer the environment immediately to give him a way to indicate "yes" and "no" and to make a choice from at least three pictures. WE also need to give him the ability to sequence information in three or four steps. These three processes promote an environment that leads to independence.

How to Assess?

Referring to your copy of the NOAH inventory, you will see a variety of ways to communicate. Simply go through the list observing and asking questions then mark down what you discover.

Which modes of communication does he use? The most commonly used are facial expressions, gestures, vocalizations, sign, words, a communication book, pictures with words, a simple device or a complex speech-generated communication device with a dynamic display.

How does he access communication? Is he vocal, or verbal? Does he access an AAC device using eye gaze, fingers/toes, hand/foot, head, single switch, two switches, keyboard, or multiple pictures on a dynamic display?

This information is particularly important to me as a speech language pathologist. Realistically, the details of what all of this means to an SLP cannot be covered in this book. However, assessing and recording this information is a good first step to helping your loved one.

Creating the environment includes how they are able to access the AAC system he needs. A speech language pathologist is the person who is required to write the report to purchase a personal AAC device. My next book will cover the use of AAC in public school systems.

What If He Can't?

Again, there is no can't. He is dependent on us to engineer the environment to create opportunities for him to use AAC. He has the right to learn how to access communication using his set of abilities.

Ways to Develop

There is more than one right way to engineer his environment. Our goal is to develop a means for him to communicate. The number one way to be successful is to provide the highest number of opportunities as possible to communicate, both receptively and expressively.

The number one way to be unsuccessful on this journey is to expect him to prove how he can use AAC that he has never been exposed to. One would think this couldn't happen. I hear this and see this every day. This leads us to Navigate.

N = Navigate (YOU CAN SEEK THE<u>N</u> FIND)
Navigate
What it Means?

Navigation means to create successful opportunities to direct, manage, and communicate. We just talked about ways to engineer his environment for communication under the prior skill. We talked about navigation earlier in the book referring to the navigator as the one who is responsible to create opportunities that have been engineered in his environment including how he accesses communication.

Navigate refers to the process of exploring different ways to use what was developed through engineering an environment that makes communication possible.

How to Assess?

Basically, you are observing how his environment has been engineered, then setting up opportunities for him to communicate as many times as possible. Too often, I observe environments where he has zero opportunities to use his AAC system to communicate. I see this regardless of age, the severity of deficits, number of years of experience the teacher or therapist possesses, or the accreditation of the school or facility.

What If He Can't?

Can't isn't an option. So far, we have set up "Together" which makes up who he is communicating with. Next, we talked about the "Hierarchy" and identifying if he is an emergent, context dependent, or independent AAC user. Following that, we learned about how to "Engineer" the environment, so others know how to communicate with him using gestures, pictures, device, etc. Now we've been learning about how to "Navigate" through his daily activities to have opportunities to communicate. It becomes easier with practice.

Ways to Develop

Earlier in this book I talked about how sometimes I will sit in the back seat of the car, so I don't have to be the navigator of the trip in the passenger seat. Guess what? You don't get to sit in the backseat ever when it comes to communication.

The opportunities have to be available so he can express himself or demonstrate that he understands whatever you just said. I find the easiest way to teach those emerging AAC skills is to have fun! The final section of the NOAH inventory is FIND. These steps lay out the ways you are going to meet all of the skills in the NOAH Program a habit for all involved!

Learning Together

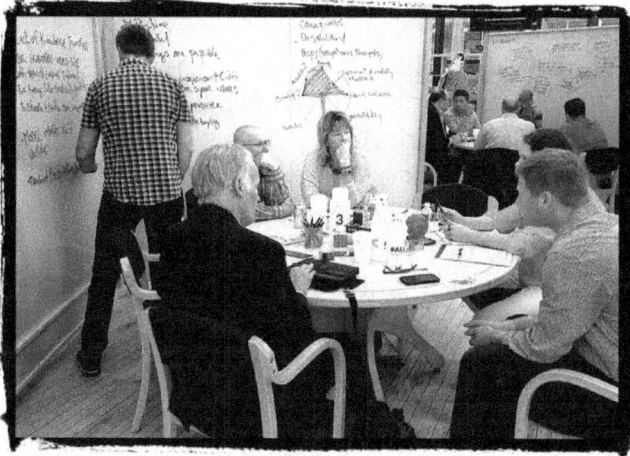

Photo courtesy of Noah's family. Edited by Paul Griesbach.

**Cynthia and Keith learning ways to help Noah
at an Assistive Technology Conference.**

Chapter 13: Step by Step: Habits for a Lifetime

Remember, YOU CAN SEEK THEN FIND.

FIND is the step-by-step process to meet the needs of the Habits for a Lifetime portion of the NOAH program.

For example, if he cannot say "I love you," you can turn the question around and ask a yes/no question. In this example, Noah answered the question with a yes! It is so important that we think of ways to get the AAC user to be able to say a message of feeling or to show that he "gets it."

Another example, instead of asking him to name all of the animals found in the jungle find a way for him to indicate that knowledge in a way in which he is can be successful. You can name five jungle animals and ask him where you find these animals. Provide him with the ability to choose between jungle, zoo, and household pets. This way he is more successful in his attempts. He has to select one picture versus five pictures. This technique works even with independent AAC users. I'm amazed at some of the techniques independent AAC users demonstrate in conversation.

NOA<u>H</u>: Habits for a Lifetime
Skill: F = Fun (YOU CAN SEEK THEN FIND)

Fun

Communication should be fun.

What it Means?

I doubt if you need a definition of what fun means so I will explain what fun has to do with communication. Fun is the component usually left out of the learning process. Successful communication is fun. It's naturally reward-driven. We learn language through movements which includes functional activity, especially play. If he wants something and he is able to communicate what he wants, he usually gets it.

Communication needs to be fast, fun, and functional. If we break those three rules, we pay for it in his lack social of skills for communication. SLPs refer to this as pragmatic language.

How to Assess?

Is his conversational turn taken in an appropriate amount of time? Is there a long pause to the point where all engaged in the conversation are bored, lost, or confused? A conversational turn must occur quickly enough to keep the conversational partner engaged in the conversation. Even if he can't take his turn quickly enough, we can help him by using pictures, recorded messages, and/or using his AAC device while speed is developed.

How do you assess fun? That's an interesting question to ask. You can assess whether the conversational turn is fast and functional, but what about fun? I work with some therapists and educators who know how to have fun! I also work with some who don't engage in fun. Fun is definitely the way to go. I'll just leave it there for now.

Is his communication functional? Can he respond to your question? Can he make a choice to indicate his desire? Can he sequence an activity or experience to communicate that message to another?

Can he stay with the topic long enough to communicate a message? I like to work up to five turns per topic. We have ways to help him learn how to do that!

Is he able to change topics instead of talking about the same topic for twenty minutes? There is only so much his conversational partner may want to hear about dinosaurs, the computer game, or even a book.

Can he end a conversation? Does he just become silent? Topic initiation, topic maintenance, and topic closure are three skills that have to be taught using AAC to make his language functional.

What If He Can't?

What if his communication isn't fun? Using all of the techniques presented in NOAH, he can learn how to communicate effectively. While you're in the navigator's seat, you have to engineer fun topics for him to interact with you or others. Focus on teaching topic initiation, maintenance, and closure.

Ways to Develop

I use a topic inventory form included with the Language Acquisition through Motor Planning (LAMP) certification manual. You can find that resource in my bibliography. It's called a topic inventory. I use this form in my consultations to help the caregiver, teacher, or therapist find some topics of interest.

Nonverbal individuals lose the natural rhythm of conversation unless someone helps them take their turn and responds to that turn. If the natural rhythm doesn't occur, that natural flow of conversation ceases. I spend much of my time reviving a natural flow of conversation. I enjoy helping others learn to improve the natural rhythm of conversation.

NOA<u>H</u>: Habits for a Lifetime
Skill: I = Independent (YOU CAN SEEK THEN FIND)

Independent

Each turn is independent.

What it Means?

Earlier in this book, I wrote in detail about the importance of taking an independent turn. This skill is present in very young children, less than six months of age; therefore, I'm not asking for something that should occur at a much later age.

Our job is to pull ourselves out of the conversation soon after initiating conversation to encourage the development of conversational independence. Avoid over prompting by allowing him to take his conversational turn by himself initially and prompt as needed. The prompt to be used the least to assist is a physical prompt.

There is a specific AAC prompting hierarchy available online. Just Google it to find the one you like.

Since so many people provide a hierarchy, I have not created one. I'll summarize briefly. On his conversational turn, the first thing the conversation partner should provide is an expectant pause which allows him to take an independent turn. If he isn't successful with that, provide an indirect verbal prompt. If still unsuccessful, request a response. Next, assist in providing a gestural cue then direct model. Finally, a physical prompt.

How to Assess?

Looking at the NOAH inventory form and answer the questions under independent.

Can he express a preferred activity using any form of communication?

Can he select a preferred activity using any form of communication?

Can he complete the "hierarchy" section with decreasing prompting, both the client and the caregiver?

Does he respond using AAC to preserve turn taking skills?

What If He Can't?

What if he isn't independent with activating switches? The first place to begin is playing with switches to activate toys, musical technology, or playing a game on a phone. When he can activate that switch or toy, begin backing yourself out of the motor interaction. Talk with him as he plays with the toy or electronic device as you would his friends who don't require assistive technology.

Ways to Develop

So how do we increase independence? Nonverbal kids and adults need us to set up communication systems for them, regardless whether the system is made up of pictures or is an advanced computer system. Once we set up the system and teach a movement or two, we need to back out of the way.

Give him a chance to explore. The number one reason he becomes dependent on another is when we don't allow him to explore. This isn't limited to communication.

Just today this mom pulled the head switch further away from the kid I was assessing so he couldn't reach the switch because he was activating the switch and playing a message his daddy had recorded. Each time he activated the switch he smiled when he heard his daddy talking. Without a doubt, he demonstrated intentional causality.

I understand that his mom removed the switch because she couldn't hear over the recorded voice. However, when kids are verbal, we have little control over what our kids choose to say or how loud they say it! Removing the switch was equivalent to taking away his voice. This promotes dependence versus independence.

Let him explore. Give him opportunities to learn to wait before he speaks. Give him a chance to be wrong. Trial and error is important in all areas of learning. Kids say the darndest things comes from exploration. This leads us to the skill of novelty.

NOA<u>H</u>: Habits for a Lifetime
Skill: N = Novel (YOU CAN SEEK THEN FIND)

Novel

Communication is original.

What it Means?

Novel means original. Being a mother of four I've heard my share of original messages my kids have said. In fact, the memory of those messages helped me embrace their adolescence. Some of the times kids say cute mispronunciations like "bambulance" for "ambulance." Sometimes they put strings of words together that aren't quite as cute.

Telling strangers, "My mommy's having a baby," when I wasn't even pregnant. If you know my eldest daughter, you know she tends to talk at the top of her lungs meaning everyone around us heard her! On many occasions, I wanted to mute her or at least lower her voice.

An error often seen with AAC whether he is learning how to use pictures or using a high-tech device is centered around vocabulary. We learn a lot from watching kids in general play. They come to us with their own expressions, their own words, and their own messages. It would be impossible to teach kids how to say every possible sentence ever uttered by humans.

This is the reason we call communication novel. Learning your ABCs and 123s is considered static learning. It's always the same; therefore, the information can be memorized. Communication is dynamic learning and it is virtually impossible to use memorized sentences as functional communication. The joy in communication comes from how it is said, not just what is said.

How to Assess?

Can he press a button to have a recorded message say a rote greeting? This is not a novel greeting. If he adds eye contact or his own personality to the greeting, it is considered novel, original. It's his.

133

Assessment of novelty almost doesn't make sense, but what you're looking for is his ability to add his own twist. Noah does not verbalize in a manner that all can understand, but I have no doubt he uses his own novel, personal, and original thoughts. Professionals just ask the family members. They can tell you what's going on!

What If He Can't?

If he isn't using novel expressions yet, use some of the items I put on the NOAH inventory under novel. Program ten novel, messages that are important to him, not just messages that everyone says. So, I'm excluding yes, no, hello, and goodbye.

Many nonverbal kids aren't using even not so original messages such as "see ya later alligator" or "after a while crocodile." Noah was tired of being offered the same cones to stack on his wheelchair tray to prove he could stack the cones. I programmed "Nope, I don't want to do this as he knocked the cones off of his tray. I'm pretty sure that was the last time that therapist placed cones on his tray. I hope.

Ways to Develop

Using all the skills in the NOAH program together helps him develop novel communication. I have no doubt about that.

I worked with a teacher who came up with the most amazing commentaries that she actually programs on her student's device for them to say. Her room is a fun place just to hang out! I'm happy to say her skills have seeped out of her classroom into the other classrooms, so things are a lot more interactive due to her work. She doesn't understand why I'm always complimenting her skills because it just comes naturally to her and her teacher assistants, but it is not common in many classrooms I visit. Unfortunately, she did not give me permission to note her comments her record her amazing skills.

NOAH: Habits for a Lifetime
Skill: D = Duplicate (YOU CAN SEEK THEN FIND)

Duplicate
Language is naturally redundant.

What it Means?
Language is naturally redundant, naturally repetitive. Let's say that again. Language is naturally redundant, naturally repetitive.

How to Assess?
Kids should be playing with the same toys repetitively. They should want to watch the same movies, hear the same songs, desire the same friends or family members. In fact, kids recite the lines to entire movies or cartoons. Is that bad in itself? I say "no." When this is looked at as a negative is when he won't watch new movies or new cartoons. He's stuck in the one script only. I'm not opening that can of worms near the end of this book. I'll save it for another book.

What If He Can't?
Encourage repetition in play. Take out a variety of toys and encourage him to do both: play over and over with the same toys *and* play with new toys. Review the nonverbal cognitive assessment portion of the NOAH inventory again if need be. Write down your findings on the NOAH inventory.

Ways to Develop
Look at your completed nonverbal cognitive assessment portion of the NOAH inventory again to find his areas of strength and weakness. You get the point. Think about any given day, the activities included in your day, the repetition naturally occurring in those activities.

One example that comes to my mind is entering passwords. Passwords alone drive me crazy. Repetition is a good thing here. If at all possible, I repeat the same password. Many, many, many years ago I would use "forget" as my password for everything I didn't think was important. I would use forget, because I would forget any other password. Of course, we "have to" change passwords every 30, 90, or 120 days so these repetitive passwords actually change but they remain repetitious. I no longer use forget because the security requirements demand more of me now.

Repetition of activities of daily living (known as ADLs) and education activities should be repetitive. Schedules and routines help him know what's occurring next. This is as true in his tooth brushing routine as it is in formal education. The NOAH program is designed to repetitive and many chapters duplicate information from another chapter in order for each chapter to stand alone in case you only have time to reach one chapter.

The inventory summary is the last portion of the Noah inventory. When I complete an assessment, I always scribble strengths, weaknesses, and goals somewhere on my test form so it only made sense to provide a spot for that important information upon on the Noah inventory.

I don't want to oversimplify the process of identifying your client or loved one's strengths, weaknesses, and goals. I'm not looking for sentence statements. I'm looking for bullets to describe his strengths such as "loves to interact", "good, sustained attention", "likes to play with toys", "enjoys looking at pictures" and/or "uses ten words". I'm looking for bullets to describe his weaknesses using statements such as "unable to say consonant sounds yet, very short attention span, doesn't explore functions of toys yet", "prefers mechanical features of toys more than the language components", or "not interested in social games".

Now that I've jotted that down, I really look at what he does well. I want to really comprehend what makes him happy, attentive, and interested in interacting with me. I look at his weaknesses and see how I can improve them by using his strengths.

Now I start to write simple goals. I write goals using the SMART method. SMART is a mnemonic to guide us in writing great goals.

S stands for Specific.
M stands for Measurable.
A stands for Attainable.
R stands for Relevant.
T stands for Time-Based.

S stands for specific. We need very specific goals. A goal such as "he will develop age-appropriate consonants of /m/, /b/, /p/, /d/, /t/ and /n/" leads us to the consonant production he currently isn't using.

"M" stands for measurable. The goal needs to be quantifiable to track progress. Goals are measured in many ways. I laugh at some goals that I've seen. 80% consistency is a commonly used measurement; however, "he will cross the street safely, 80% of opportunities" does not help him much. We have to think about how we can picture that goal being achieved. I want to see that he can produce the above consonants. In this goal, I'm looking at his ability to produce the consonant in isolation. I want to see the presence of these consonant sounds in his daily routines. Later I will add goals to combine those consonants with vowels and other consonants

"A" stands for attainable which means your goal is realistic and you have the tools or the ability of attaining those tools through therapy or home programs to achieve that goal. I believe that both kids and adults should always be working on their ability to produce these sounds; therefore, using his lips and tongue in some manner is attainable. This does not mean that all individuals will have intelligible speech. That's why we develop other goals as well. Utilization of AAC is a must.

"R" stands for Relevant. This means that your goal has something to do with your overall mission. I want him to communicate so my goals will be linked directly to communication.

137

"T" stands for Time-Based. Your goal has a deadline. Although speech pathologists like the use of open-ended questions, goals need to be close-ended. All goals must have the date it is determined to be achieved. I write annual goals but will add new goals whenever a goal is achieved.

Congratulations you have completed the Noah inventory and are ready to implement a program. I am available to help you through this process. Please contact me through my website **Lv2pla.com** or my email lpgriesbach@gmail.com.

Don't Wait for All the Answers, just Live and Make Your Own Fun

"Professionals are too busy

debating each other over what works

while families live today."

Chapter 14: How His Family Filled the Gap

I'm including this chapter to share my personal thoughts and passion. One thing we older people can agree on is time changes. Ideas come and go until we're back where we started.

CPR certification is just one example. I've been recertified every year or two since I was seventeen. The techniques and processes go back and forth. I guess that's why we have to get certified so often. I was actually taught a new way to wash my hands during orientation with a newly contracted job.

Other things change too such as how frequently or infrequently we wash our hair, our bodies, our laundry. How often we change the oil in our vehicles. The standards our kids are taught and tested on change too.

I'm writing this entry from a campsite. My husband Paul and I choose to rough it in our SUV. Most wouldn't choose similar sleeping quarters. As I look around the campground, I see tents, pop ups, trailers, motorhomes, fifth wheelers, and one of the latest sleeping hammocks. All of these are great ideas for someone, but not everyone. In fact, many would say thanks, but no thanks. Some of you would even say no to the campground and head to the Hilton. We all decide what's fun in our lives.

Those living in the nonverbal community aren't stopping their lives waiting on "professionals" to figure fun out for them. Cynthia and Keith, Noah's parents, brought him home shortly after birth thinking everything was okay. They believed everything about Noah was okay. They were happy with their new addition to their family of four. They had plans for Noah's future like we all do for our children. It would be months or years before they knew they were on a different journey. Knowing Cynthia's and Keith's personalities, I don't believe for a moment that they stopped and did nothing.

I have been blessed through the years to see how many families of kids with special needs power through their journey. They don't sit and wait on us professionals to plan their day. They wake up every morning, after an unrestful night in most situations, to start their day. I always tell the moms, dads, siblings, grandparents, or other caregivers I work with that they are the ones that make the difference in their kid's life.

Professionals are too busy debating each other over what works while the families are living today. Sounds harsh, but I do place blame on professionals: therapists, doctors, specialists, nurses, teachers, counselors, etc. We have this idea of "proof" forced down our throats so frequently and intensely that we are in a waiting mode for the magical answers.

I won't wait. I haven't waited. I explore and look at what seems to work. I also listen. I listen to the clients with whom I get the privilege to work daily. I listen to the moms, dads, grandparents, siblings, teachers and all others involved in his life. I pay attention to the research. I read books from long ago, the stuff that had meaning and wasn't dependent on a computer. I also read the new stuff. I'm very analytical and am continuously learning from multiple sources.

Let's talk about what is working that parents have shared with me or I've observed with my own eyes.

Go on trips.

Noah's family is a great example for this. They have a very loved van adapted for Noah's wheelchair and even a place for an adult to sleep in back. They aren't afraid to take a nurse along with them or to be the nursing staff all by themselves. They research places that Noah could enjoy and whether there are enough adaptations to make it a fun experience for Noah. They have taken Noah to Florida to the amusement parks and to Chicago to see the Cubs play.

These are long journeys, but they also visit many places in the community. They attend family get-togethers in local restaurants. Both Cynthia and Keith are explorers so this fits their personalities. If you aren't an explorer, you may not venture on a fifteen-hour drive and spend all the energy it takes to figure out the journey.

That's ok. Be you. Research your area and find things your family can enjoy. This may be joining a support group to find out the activities scheduled in your local area. I don't tell parents to do this. I'm just sharing ideas that I've observed families doing. For some, just going to Chik-Fil-a is an enjoyable outing. Right, Evan?

Expect him to talk.

I can't cover this area without talking about Evan's mom. Felicia has retained her natural instincts as a mom when it comes to teaching communication, activities, family, etc. Evan is vocal and able to work on speaking because she never lost the expectation that he should speak to people. I'll admit it is sometimes painful to watch Evan try to verbalize, but it's worth it in the end. Evan is talking even though unfamiliar listeners cannot fully understand him. Who cares? His family understands him. He is able to participate in articulation therapy with me because of verbal expectations and he knows how to speak.

Have parties and playdates.

I am so grateful to the families that keep this in mind. Often these dates include a bonus for the adults involved as they chat with the play date's parent(s). I see this done just over coffee or on a large scale. Cynthia and Keith hosted the Purple Ball several years ago to promote epilepsy awareness and to give the kids a chance to wear formal dresses and suits. All of us adults dressed formally too. It was amazing!

Keep your eyes on their peers.

Pay attention to what his peers are doing. What's age appropriate? This helps you transition out of baby topics and move him along the journey. Caution: Try not to waste time comparing levels of development. It's easier for me to write this than do, but it is futile and takes away time you could be doing something more rewarding. I mention this only because

Noah has had teachers read him preschool rhymes and books instead of something more related to his age level.

Take a day off.

Give yourself and your child a day off. Stay in pajamas all day. Do what is fun for you and your family. Do only what needs to be done. These breaks lead you into a better tomorrow.

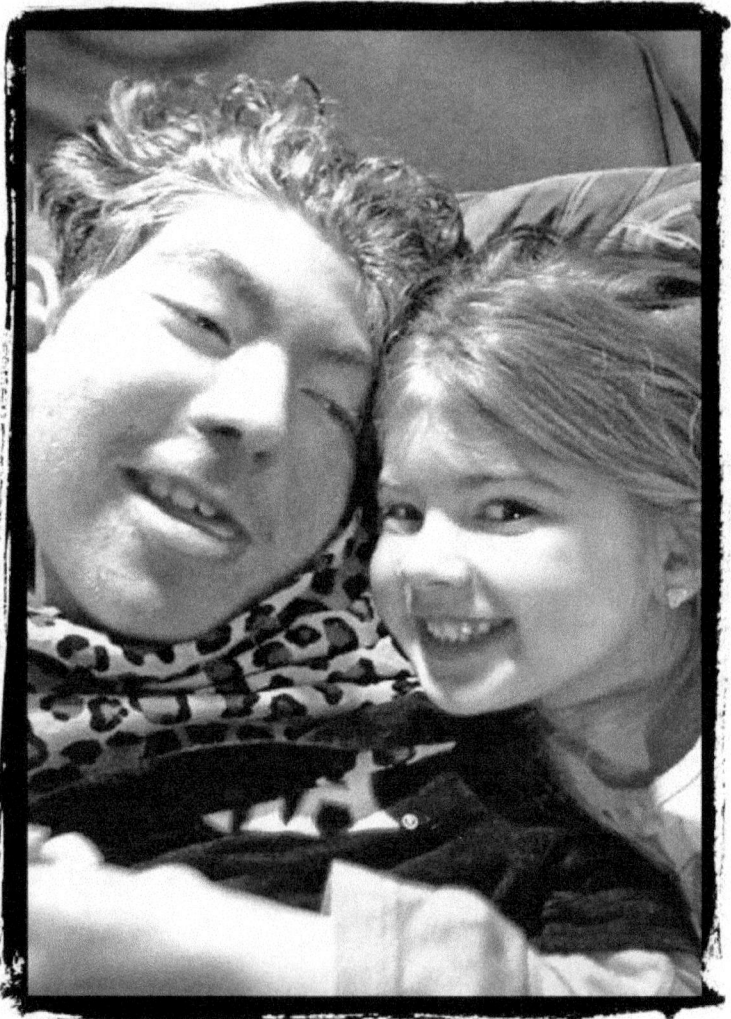

Photo courtesy of Noah's family. Edited by Paul Griesbach.

Kinlee knows just what to do for Noah.

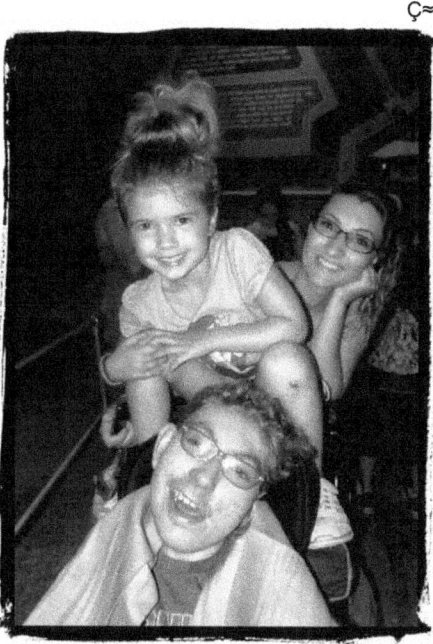

Tristan and Kinlee are just what Noah has needed.

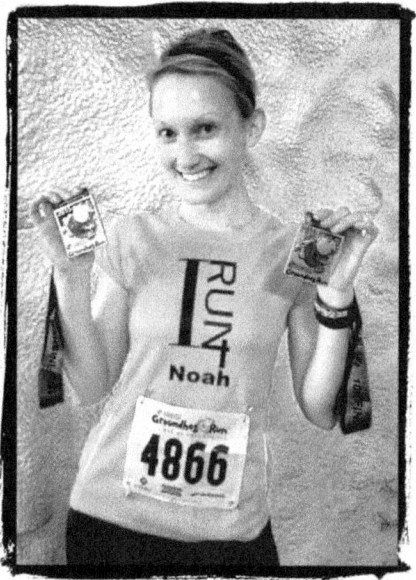

Sarah runs for Noah.

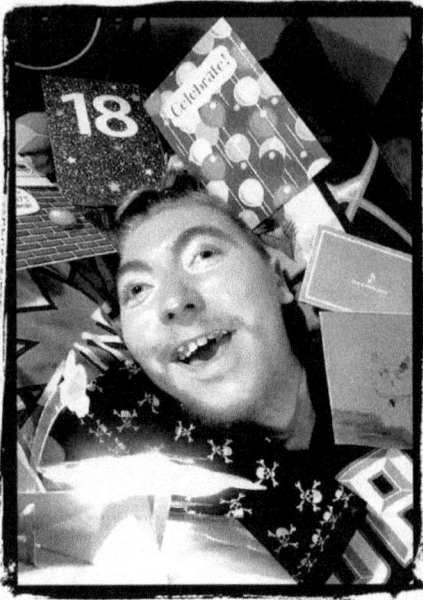

**Noah's annual birthday
card competition.
He is trying to get one from
each state and as many countries
as possible.**

**Keith and Cynthia Mosley
figured out pool access
on their own.**

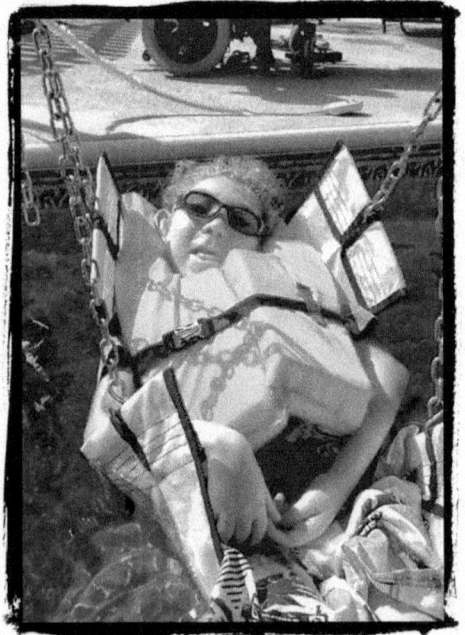

Photos courtesy of Noah's family. Edited by Paul Griesbach.

146

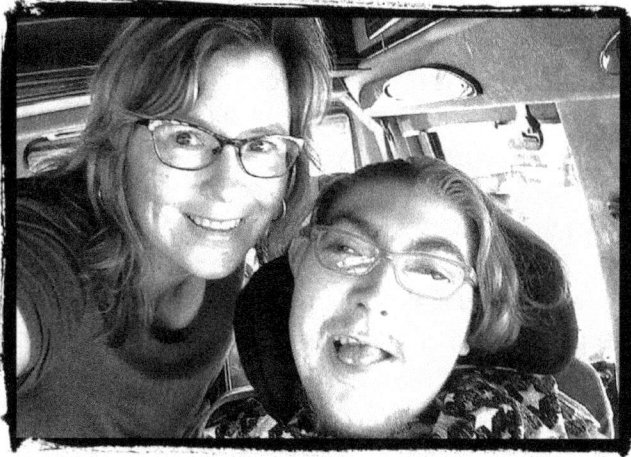

Cynthia and Noah drive miles in their van for adventures.

We've Got This!

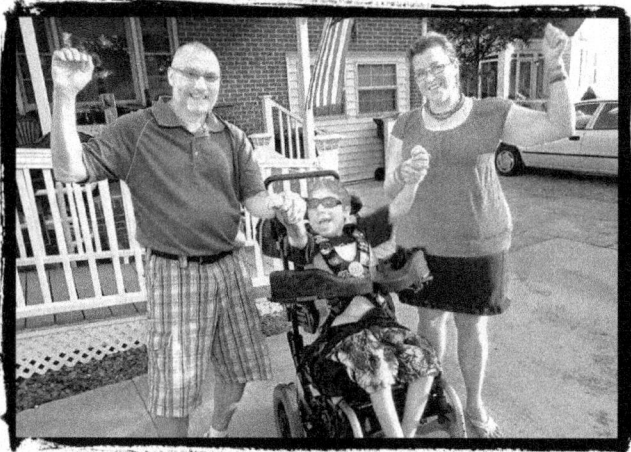

Noah and his wonderful parents, Keith and Cynthia.

Photos courtesy of Noah's family. Edited by Paul Griesbach.

Chapter 15:
For the Caregiver

This chapter is for you, the caregiver, to help you begin the journey to communication. I've tried to simplify complex information throughout this book to help you. I'm aware of the unfamiliar terms which complicate it all the more. I want you to see that help is available for you and your loved one(s). There are professionals and paraprofessionals out there to help you.

That being said, I want you to know that you're the boss. That's right, you are the boss. You are the caregiver, the one who makes essential daily decisions for him.

After the professionals and paraprofessionals come into your life, things get complicated quickly. You may become overwhelmed and give control over to them to make the decisions we need to help you make.

I want you to know that as the parents, the guardians, the spouse, the grandparents, etc. you are the ones to research the information presented, then make a choice or choices of intervention. I know it's complicated. I also know there is no magic cure to make your loved one talk in a day.

I do know that as you build your team, you are also developing a support system. Refer to the list your created on the NOAH inventory for the AAC in the THEN section of YOU CAN SEEK *THEN* FIND. Who did you list as your team? What role do these people play on your team? How do they make life hopeful? How do they help you make the tough decisions?

My goal for writing the NOAH program is for you to build a team that you lead as the caregiver. Each individual on the team should be providing you information within their area of expertise. In turn, you take all of that information and apply it to each area of his life. I feel like my job is to help you do this. I assist you in ways to help you understand what I'm teaching you and how to work that step–by- step process into your day.

As a SLP I glean information about your loved one's comprehensive development and how those skills work together. All team members can change the day-to-day activities, but we are all moving forward to facilitate communication.

By using the NOAH program, you are working simultaneously with your team to improve cognitive and language skills, oral motor skills, and giving him a means to communicate. You are finding ways to incorporate these habits into your daily routines.

Just Ask

"I spend more time training caregivers

and paraprofessionals than

professionals

because they ask me."

Chapter 16:
Take the Next Step

This chapter is a bit more technical. Although, it is directed toward professionals to get them moving in the right direction, to help the kids on their caseload or the ones who should be on their caseload, I never leave caregivers out. I spend more time helping caregivers and paraprofessionals than I do teachers and therapists because you ask for my help.

I know a lot of the information in this book is new, or at least a new way of looking at it. It was written to fill the gaps of what is currently available. I have provided you with the resources to go to work tomorrow and initiate NOAH now. I'm aware it is a lot of information and you are amongst the grassroots effort to follow an actual step by step program to help your nonverbal clients or loved one(s). In addition to this book when I present the NOAH program, I always suggest that you use the accompanying NOAH inventory which is currently available during my presentations or on my website Lv2Pla.com. It really does make it easier to "get this" so you can use it right away.

I provide NOAH consults to assess nonverbal cognitive skills, oral motor function skills related to swallowing/speech production and develop an AAC system for your loved one.

Let's talk a little about AAC. AAC is complex. It's not natural. You will require assistance to identify which system(s) will work and how to use AAC. You will find many different approaches to the process. You are probably wondering why I said that. I say that because I'm honest. Time and money are required for intervention. Deciphering different approaches and communication devices is also a part of it. It's kind of like buying a mattress these days – so many kinds and you don't really know how well it will work for you until you try it. Just like a mattress, there are different options to explore.

Let me give you another example. I enjoy training service dogs. Service dogs are nothing more than assistive technology. I look at training service dogs from two points-of-view when training the people holding the leash and training the dog. One perspective is from the viewpoint of the individual training the dog initially for the person who needs the service dog. The other perspective comes from the handler, the person who requires the service dog.

The trainer trains the dog and prepares the dog to work for the person needing the service dog. The next step is when the trainer decreases their authority on the dog allowing the person needing the services of the dog to "handle" the dog.

It's very similar with AAC. As the trainer, you guide your child in the use of the AAC device. This means you will need to learn how to use and program the device. You will set it up with the messages your child will require in order to communicate. Next, you will be teaching him how to use the communication device and how to program the device. You are still there every day to assist but your prompting will decrease in order for your child to become an independent AAC user. The step-by-step process will help you become proficient as the trainer and your loved one as the AAC user.

Further training of NOAH is available through consultations, face-to-face presentation, webinars and recordings. Rome wasn't built in a day, neither is communication.

Pull out your NOAH inventory to get started. Complete the inventory. Write down his strengths. Write down his weaknesses. Develop goals to strengthen his weaknesses.

SMART Goals

Write SMART goals so you can see him achieve his goals. SMART goals are:
S: Specific
M: Measurable
A: Attainable
R: Relevant
T: Time-bound.
Once his goals are achieved, repeat the process again and master new goals. Remember you are always working on nonverbal cognitive skills, oral motor skills, AAC, and developing daily habits to improve his communication to last a lifetime.

Thank you for taking the time to read *NOAH: The Best Gift Ever – A Voice for Everyone.* I hope this book has helped you grow on your journey down the nonverbal communication path. Please let me know how I can help you on your journey.

Quick Reference

The NOAH program is an innovative, four-pronged approach designed by Laura Phillips Griesbach, M.S., CCC-SLP to give you the tools to help those who are unable to speak gain a voice. The program uses two mnemonic devices to help guide you. The name NOAH and the phrase YOU CAN SEEK THEN FIND.

NOAH

N = Nonverbal cognitive assessment
O = Oral motor intervention
A = Another means to communicate
H = Developing habits to generalize

YOU

Y = You do (Imitation/copying sounds and actions)
O = Object Permanence (the necessary skill of knowing an object exists even when the object is out of sight)
U = Understanding (directions and questions)

CAN

C = Cause-effect (action equals reaction)
A = A means to an end (using available skills to get what is needed)
N = Needs met (use of any communication to convey what is desired)

SEEK

S =Sensory (the body's response to input)
E = Examine (body posture, position, and movement)
E = Explore (mouth movement)
K = Kinesiology (muscle movement)

THEN

T = Together (who he interacts with)
H = Hierarchy (there is an order to development)
E = Engineer (create the environment)
N = Navigate (create successful opportunities)

FIND

F = Fun (communication should be fun)
I =Independent (each person has a turn)
N = Novel (communication is original)
D = Duplicate (language is naturally redundant)

About the Author

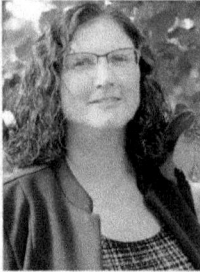

Laura Phillips Griesbach has served as a Speech Language Pathologist for infants through geriatrics since 1989. Laura is passionate about working with those who need her most. Specializing in communication, Laura provides new insight for clients who have suffered brain trauma whether at birth or at the age of 103. Constant motion and deep analysis is where Laura spends her time. Always seeking the way to help a client, student, colleague, caregiver, allied professional, physician, educator, or elected government official to grow is what truly fuels Laura's passion.

With personal growth in mind, Laura joined the John Maxwell Team to become a certified speaker, coach, and trainer. Laura offers professional workshops, seminars, keynote speaking, coaching and therapeutic consultation through her practice, LV2PLA, which stands for Love to Play. Laura continues to play with infants on the floor or adults at the table to facilitate communication skills for a lifetime. Her passion is to help others grow to meet their goals.

She considers herself blessed to have so many opportunities to guide individuals through the process in order to help leaders maximize their effectiveness, to help caregivers restore wholeness to individuals in their family following severe illness or trauma, and to communicate and advocate for those who can't speak, yet.

She advocates at the state and national level to change awareness in medical and educational institutions. Although change is slow, she is committed to helping others realize that communication is a right, not just a privilege! Laura has broadened her goals, founded LV2PLA, and achieved certification by JMT to specialize in personal and professional growth.

When Laura isn't deep in thought, you can find her with her husband hiking and camping. She enjoys spending time with her children and grandchildren. Dogs add joy to her life. She lives in a rural community outside of Richmond, Virginia.

Laura would love to hear from you and learn about your experiences with the NOAH program and your journey toward empowering others to throw away the phrases "he can't" or "I don't know what do" and start making progress toward freeing their love one today. She can be reached to share your experiences or schedule a training in your area through her website **Lv2Pla.com** or email **lpgriesbach@gmail.com**

Acknowledgements

I can't even begin to list or adequately show my appreciation to all who have helped the NOAH program become more than just a jumble of ideas in my head into a viable program with a website and now even a book or maybe a series of books. NOAH is already helping people gain more freedom and independence and I am immensely grateful for all who accompanied me on this journey.

First, as I noted in the dedication, I am eternally grateful to Noah and his wonderful parents, Cynthia and Keith.

I also owe gratitude to all the excellent teachers, mentors and clinical supervisors I had along the way including Dr. Eileen Abrahamsen at Old Dominion University, Dr. Claire Waldron and Mrs. Beverly Crouse from Radford University.

And, of course my family and friends who listened to me talk about this endlessly for years and who helped by reading rough, rough, rough drafts and helping transform it into just a rough draft and finally an edited piece.

I owe gratitude to my husband, Paul. Paul has helped me through the many steps of publishing this book. Paul has designed my website. He helped with the edits, the graphics, the woes of technology, and especially the photography which is seen on the cover and throughout the book. Paul is writing a series of Little Paul books to help bring literacy into children's life. Paul has allowed me to develop age-appropriate phonological processing and AAC features into these books for those learning to read. I'm fortunate to have him on this adventure called life with me.

Special thanks to my colleague Michelle Alexander Warner, OTR and my sister, Shelly Murphy who is a professional writer and editor. These two were not afraid to tell me what I needed to hear and to move and even delete whole sections of the book to make it clearer and more concise. If there's any part that still isn't clear, it's on me. Their red pens and red tracking notes were well honed and precise.

Description

You are picking up a book which empowers to give the gift of communication to those whom are trapped within their own thoughts.

Due to autism, verbal apraxia, traumatic brain injury, cerebral palsy, aphasia, epilepsy, dysarthria, Parkinson's, multiple sclerosis, ALS, vascular dementia, Down syndrome etc. many children and adults remain nonverbal and are unable to communicate their thoughts.

Now you have the information to learn and apply today! Make the difference for your loved one and/or client using a four-pronged approach designed for success.

Develop the skills to unlock communication using the NOAH program which combines a nonverbal cognitive assessment and treatment plan, oral motor intervention to develop verbal skills, acquire another means to communicate using AAC, and develop cognitive and communication skills to last a lifetime! Welcome to our journey!

Book Review

Laura is an amazing SLP with a huge heart and undeniable passion to find any available means to tap into a clients' abilities to give a voice to those who are otherwise viewed as locked in. Her passion and drive is contagious and her method is thorough, yet simplified and concise for implementation by loved ones, paraprofessionals, or professionals.

Her NOAH Inventory checklist provides a great reference for guidance with implementing the step-by-step mnemonic for the entire assessment process to determine patient abilities and their means for communication. Laura's method provides the inspiration & tools to help connect with clients who are typically viewed as unreachable and would otherwise fall through the cracks.

-   Michelle Alexander Warner, OTR

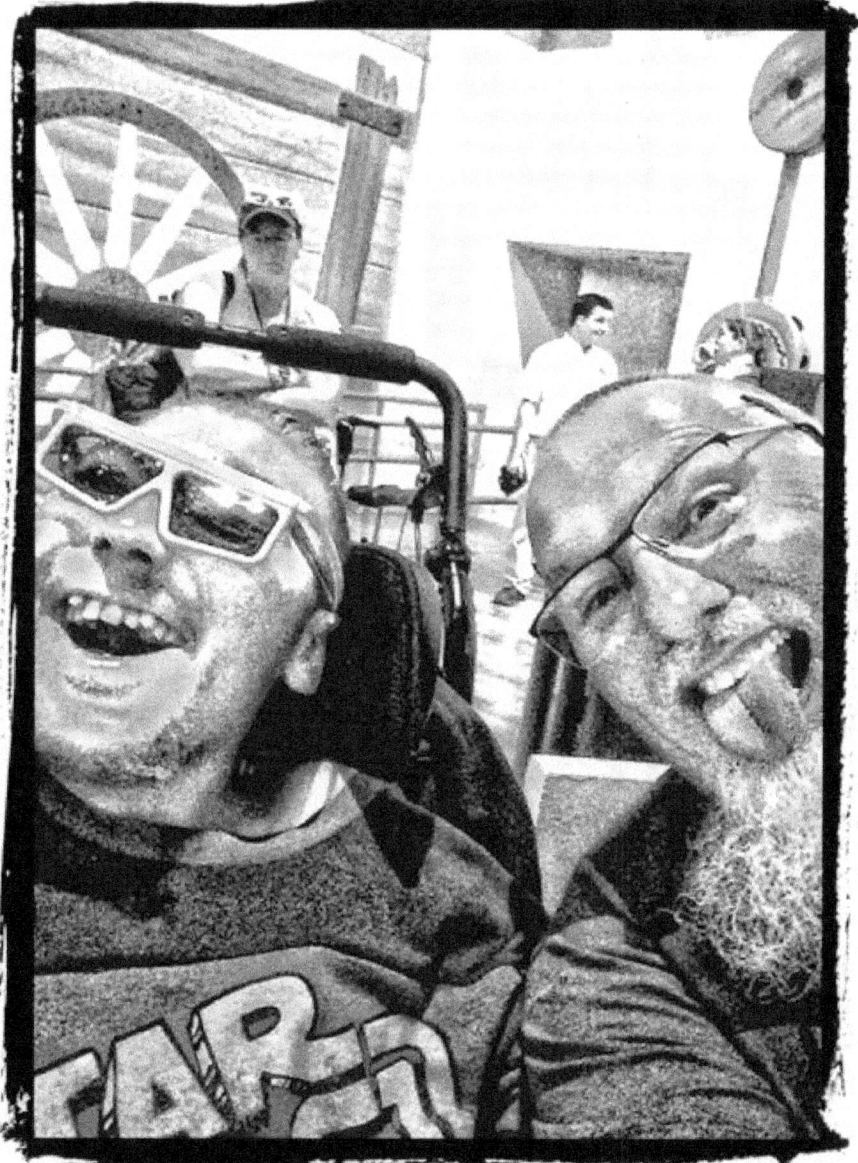

Photo courtesy of Noah's family. Edited by Paul Griesbach.

Noah and his dad, Keith, love Star Wars and Disney.

161

www.ingramcontent.com/pod-product-compliance
Lightning Source LLC
LaVergne TN
LVHW052027080426
835513LV00018B/2193